Individuals, Householders, Citizens

Individuals, Householders, Citizens

Malayalis and Family Planning, 1930–1970

J. DEVIKA

zubaan

Individuals, Householders, Citizens:
Malayalis and Family Planning, 1930–1970
by J. Devika
Published (2008) by
ZUBAAN
an imprint of Kali for Women
K-92, 1st Floor
Hauz Khas Enclave
NEW DELHI - 110 016
Email: zubaanwbooks@vsnl.net and zubaan@gmail.com
Website: www.zubaanbooks.com

First Published (2008) by Zubaan

10 9 8 7 6 5 4 3 2 1

ISBN-13: 978-81-89884-47-5
ISBN-10: 81-89884-47-6

Zubaan is an independent feminist publishing house based in New Delhi, India, with a strong academic and general list. It was set up as an imprint of the well known feminist house Kali for Women, and carries forward Kali's tradition of publishing world quality books to high editorial and production standards. "Zubaan" means tongue, voice, language, speech in Hindustani. Zubaan is a non-profit publisher, working in the areas of the humanities, social sciences, as well as in fiction, general non-fiction, and books for young adults that celebrate difference, diversity and equality, especially for and about the children of India and South Asia under its imprint Young Zubaan.

Typset at Tulika Print Communication Services
35 A/1, (3rd Floor), Shahpur Jat, New Delhi - 110 049
Printed at Brijbasi Art Press Ltd., E-46/11, Okhla Industrial Area, PH-II, New Delhi - 110 020

Contents

Acknowledgements

Coming to the end of a book-length work is so like coming to the end of an exciting, if exhausting, journey. One cannot help looking back and re-learn, once again, the lesson of humility. At this moment, the small and large kindnesses, from people far and near, which have made the journey possible, come into full view.

The kindnesses I have benefited from are indeed many, and varied. The research for this book was funded by the Kerala Research Programme on Local-level Development, Centre for Development Studies, Thiruvananthapuram. Dr K N Nair, who headed it, provided me ample support, notwithstanding his early misgivings about the feasibility of this inquiry. Then, soon, I found lasting friendships there: Christopher, who was always cheerful, because of whom I remained unintimidated by paperwork; Dr P R Gopinathan Nair, the most patient listener imaginable; and Vineetha Menon, who became my best reader and one of my dearest friends; Dr K N Raj and Dr K K Subramanian who were very encouraging, at crucial moments. Later, CDS provided me with the opportunities to present the early drafts of chapters through which I was able to sharpen and clarify these ideas. I thank Dr Michael Tharakan for his careful reading and criticism, but even more for being such an unbelievably generous source of information and inspiration. Mala Ramanathan, who provided incisive comments on a chapter, was also instrumental in provoking me into undertaking this research; Uday and Mala have remained major sources of encouragement. Several scholars and friends—

Dr Mohan Rao, K.T. Rammohan, Praveena Kodoth, Judith Heyer, Ruchi Chaturvedi, Paul Zachariah, S Irudaya Rajan, Fillippo and Caroline Osella, Sundari Ravindran, Sharmila Sreekumar, and especially Vineetha Menon—took the trouble of reading the draft chapters. Of all my readers, I thank Dr Mohan Rao the most. He graciously read and commented on my half-done chapters, urged me to polish, polish, and repolish the arguments, and also cautioned me to beware of the 'French School of Obscure Writing'! If this book has any clarity, that is surely the result of the efforts of my readers, while all the errors are certainly mine. Other friends made life colourful when it threatened to turn a dull and tenebrous gray. I do not know how to thank Praveena, Sreedevi, Narayanan, Beena, Gilbert, Ambili/Pulari, Shajahan, Anindita, Gouridasan, Vineetha, Dilip Raj, Sajitha, Mini, Anitha, and Usha. Without Usha's constant support, I would have missed out on a lot of reading: I can't thank her enough. Neesar *maash* continues to remain the single largest inspiration not only for this, but also for everything I write. Sanjeev helped me to polish the writing further.

Thanks are also due to the staff of the libraries in Thiruvananthapuram, Kottayam, Thrissur, and Kozhikode, who often went beyond their normal routines to help me. Binumol Abraham, my research assistant, was always cheerful, patient, and encouraging.

At home, Radhamani Chechi helped me to keep up with the normal hum of domestic and school routines; she has been my refuge in ways she herself may not have realized. Sreekutty and Kunhammu, who fill my life with love and laughter, have contributed to this book through a thousand little sacrifices that cannot be weighed on adult-scales. My brothers, and also our large extended family, which keeps my life warm and cosy, have always been proud supporters of my work. My mother, Dr C Jayakumari, who passed away before this work was fully done, was always concerned that I work too much, is fondly remembered. This book, however, is dedicated to my beloved grandaunt, Ratna Bai, whose memory will continue to illumine every day of my life.

Introduction

Pride and Patriarchy

As a child growing up amidst the vast expansion of public discussion around development in Kerala in the 1970s and 80s, my sense of being Malayali was shaped by the claim that we were, as a people, more 'socially developed' than other Indians. This, I vaguely felt, made us slightly superior to fellow-Indians. The fact that we had a certain distinct linguistic and cultural identity was also important; yet, in the din raised about social development, it seemed less decisive. In the 1970s especially I dimly understood that we were somehow poorer than many parts of India, especially metropolitan areas, from where my cousins came home for holidays. We consumed much less of everything in those days than they did. However, 'social development' seemed to make up for that: our social development was the guarantee of our moral and intellectual superiority. We were 'civilized' and 'socially advanced'; we could be proud.

I entered adulthood in times when the celebrated 'Kerala Model'—high degrees of social development occurring with low levels of economic growth[1]—began to be increasingly problematized, and not only by those at its margins. While excluded sections of people protested against their exclusion, those who were included—including myself, as an upper-caste, upper-class, educated young woman—protested against the almost-unbreachable forms of regulation that subserved entrenched gender hierarchies, which were no less than the conditions for inclusion. It was clear by now that the production of knowledge on social development in Kerala did not serve academic or policy purpose alone. Kerala has always been of interest to anthropologists, primarily because of matriliny. In the mid-twentieth century political scientists took deep interest in Malayali communism. Social scientific research within Kerala in the 1980s was not remarkably vibrant with the exception of not very surprisingly, development studies and allied disciplines like demography. Development was at the focus of social scientific research concerns, and this continues today, to some degree. However, the problematization of the 'Kerala Model' made it amply evident that such knowledge also shaped the very ideological underpinnings of being a 'modern Malayali'. In the 1980s and 1990s, the mobilizations challenging entrenched notions of development around issues of marginalized groups such as tribals, dalits, and the fisherfolk, and around gender power, exerted such pressure that this ideological construct, the 'modern Malayali', is now bursting at the seams. Critical work on the claims of social development in Kerala is proliferating in the present, in a variety of disciplinary and political orientations.

This work participates in the continuing critique of the 'Kerala Model', and seeks to unravel the particular ways in which people were interpellated into the discourse of family planning. The focus therefore, is on how people were prepared for inclusion. I have found this route particularly useful for two reasons. First, it moves beyond an exclusive focus on the assessment of outcomes, which is by now a route preferred by many critics of Kerala's achievements. Pointing to the differential gains made by social groups is certainly crucial; however, this does not often tell us how inclusions and exclusions, which resulted in such outcomes, were instituted and perpetuated. Secondly, it moves beyond an exclusive focus on exclusion. Such a view prevents us from seeing that those who were included were themselves subjected to distinct forms of regulation within specific regimes of power, which too need to be recognized and critiqued. This of course does not mean that the exclusions will be forgotten. The focus is not on capturing the empirical outcomes. The discursive processes by which the inclusions/exclusions are effected will be at the heart of this work.

The explorations undertaken here centre around the broader socio–historical processes that shaped the popular acceptance of artificial contraception in Kerala, which I locate in the decades between 1930 and 1970. The early public debates on the desirability of contraception began around the early 1930s. The first successful mass vasectomy camp at Ernakulam, in which thousands of men were sterilized, and an event celebrated in the popular press as a major development achievement, occurred in 1970.[2] Reflecting as a relatively privileged Malayali woman on the ambiguities of the 'liberation' attributed to us as a class by the proponents of the Kerala Model, I was amazed by some striking mismatches. Particularly by the mismatches between the shrill claims relating to women's agency, contraception-acceptance, and the 'progressiveness' of modern Malayali society, and the embarrassment that cloaked sex and contraception in everyday discourse. Malayalis continue to be largely silent on contraception—full contraceptive information remains largely inaccessible to young and unmarried, and often, married women. Thus while the celebration of family planning in population control, family welfare, and maternal health, even today, is conducted at a deafeningly high pitch, the very possibility of using contraception to widen women's choices (viewed as distinct from those that contribute to the upward mobility of families), seems weakly projected. Also, 'legitimate' sex seems confined to marriage, and contraceptive information appears to need no further spread. It almost seemed as though the Malayali exceptionalism—the image of Kerala as a progressive society—worked to make invisible the new forms of patriarchy that mediated our lives. Recent research into women's health in Kerala confirms many of these observations. It has, for instance, been pointed out recently that the celebration of women's better reproductive health in Kerala masks a number of worrying features, both already existent, and newly emergent, of their health-seeking behaviour[3] (Sowmini and Sarma 2004; Mishra 2006).

It must be noted that the non-coerced acceptance of contraception (or family planning) by the masses in Kerala is frequently hailed as a major element in Kerala's achievement of

'Model' status.[4] This is often read as implicitly indicating a 'higher' political consciousness or a greater capacity for rational choice (for instance, Jeffrey 2003). In this case, we have no further reason to investigate the history of state-centred contraception provision; all we have to do is to prevent the deterioration of achieved levels. On closer inspection, however, it is often conceded that there are undesirable aspects: for instance, women in Kerala seem to have borne a disproportionately large share of the burdens of contraception,[5] yet these have not provoked much critical inspection of the history of contraception in Kerala. At best, they are acknowledged to be serious issues which, however, merely mean that some aspects of irrationality, eminently exterminable, have succeeded in surviving. The demographic literature foregrounds the acceptance of birth control in Kerala as rational choice under given circumstances. For my purposes, however, this says too little. So, how do we understand the transformation of rural life in Kerala as an element in the heightened preference for small families? Consider this answer: the twentieth century, on one hand, saw the rise of new aspirations among more and more sections of the people; on the other, economic opportunities for their realization remained dismally low. This gave rise to a situation in which birth control became a rational strategy for upward mobility. When demography aspires merely to be a policy science, it can stop at this. However, in order to understand the relations of power that inured in such transformations, we may have to look more carefully at the notions of respectability and the good life emergent in Malayali modernity. We may have to see what kinds of hierarchies they presupposed, what kinds of élitism they authorized, and how these mediated the attitudes and access of different social groups to contraceptive services. The persistence of narrow developmentalist commonsense ensures that the larger socio–historical conditions within which Malayalis limited births remain clouded.[6] One, then, has no means of examining whether and how this choice is bound up with the emergence of new forms of power, new gendered subjectivities, institutions and hierarchies, within which these choices are made. When the apparently power-neutral 'enlightened rationality' is seen to be directing the spread of the nuclear family-form and the small family in mid-twentieth century Kerala, the crucial emergence of the new patriarchy that underpinned the modern patrifocal nuclear family is obscured. The rhetoric of choice also blurs the changing forms of power that binds the state and society within which these options unfold.

Seeking ways of thinking through these issues, I have been deeply influenced by contemporary global debates on development, political power, and the feminist debates on birth control and bodily autonomy. The new interdisciplinary work on questions traditionally considered native to demography alone became another major inspiration. Besides, recent critical literature on Kerala's development, critiques of health and health care in India from social medicine, and expanding work on the history of birth control in India too frame this exercise. Some more detail about these in the following section.

The Context and the Inspirations

First, this work is located within an academic context in which development is being interrogated with such unprecedented thoroughness that its self-evidence has been severely weakened (Ferguson 1990; Escobar 1995; Cowen and Shenton 1996). Indeed, the economism, the Eurocentrism, and the teleological social evolutionism that has underpinned the many variants of development discourse—Modernization Theory, Marxism—is no longer fashionable. Nor are the claims of political modernization—about the secular and popular grounding of state power, about the continuous expansion of citizenship—uncritically taken. Cross-cultural comparisons, too are not accepted to be culturally neutral; rather they are recognized as actively implicated in the processes by which inclusions and exclusions occur. This enables, too, a critical distancing from the self-claims of 'social development' which do not centralize economic growth but share many of the basic features of developmentalism, especially Eurocentrism and teleology.

Secondly, this has also been shaped to a very considerable degree by the recent discussions on the nature of governmental power and its implications for state power and development that have accrued around Michel Foucault's conceptualization of the political rationality of government (Foucault 1988). Talal Asad has argued that:

> Within the modern world which has come into being, changes have taken place as the effect of dominant political power by which new possibilities are constructed and old ones destroyed. The changes do not reflect a simple expansion of the range of individual choice, but the creation of conditions in which only new (i.e. modern) choices can be made. The reason for this is that the changes involve the re-formation of subjectivities and the reorganization of social spaces in which subjects act and are acted upon. The modern state—imperial, colonial, post-colonial—has been crucial to these processes of construction/destruction. (Asad 1992: 337)

One of the common threads that run through all varieties of reformist discourse under colonialism and after—the colonial official's, the missionary's, the newly-educated local élite's, the post-colonial developmental activist's—is the strident differentiation of 'progress' from 'ignorance/superstition', and the faith that the latter may be alleviated by rooting out the material, social, and ideological conditions in which it thrives. Thus, far from 'liberating' subjects into a neutral realm of 'choices', such reformist projects sought, to eliminate the basic nurturing conditions of 'undesirable' traits. This would radically alter the significance granted to civil society and the nascent public sphere (both of which were emergent under colonial conditions in the late nineteenth century) within the still-dominant views of the modern history of Kerala. This would signify not so much the expansion of free will, unfettered rational public debate, or autonomous agency, as the construction of a space for the operation of modern political rationality—which is *governmental*. The government of individuals involves the deployment of a form of power that aims at getting individuals to act and commit themselves to ends projected in general models of possible action (Burchell et al. 1991). This presupposes and calls for freedom and capacity for activity, and also reasonableness, on the part of the governed. The public sphere, then, may be viewed as a space in which modern power operates, with disruption, subversion, and contestation, precisely through the construction of ostensibly 'free' and 'autonomous' subjectivities. In Malayali society, the emergence of the project and problem of attaining a balance between totalizing power and an individualizing power to achieve the government of individuals has been central to discussions around the notion of society and power since the late nineteenth century. This understanding frames the historical inquiry undertaken here.

Thirdly, this work explores (some of) the possibilities opened up by recent work in anthropological and historical demography, which displays extraordinary sensitivity towards the role of cultural change in mediating such large-scale changes as the demographic transition. The interdisciplinary turn in the social sciences has certainly not left demography untouched: in the past two decades, creative exchanges between demographers, cultural anthropologists, and historians have highlighted the importance of the changing meanings of procreation, family life, and the good life, in understanding changes in fertility[7] (Caldwell et al. 1987; Carter 1988; Basu and Aaby 1988; McLaren 1990; Kertzer 1992; Greenhalgh 1995). This has broken down the disciplinary and methodological boundaries that continue to work within the dominant literature on the Malayali fertility transition. For instance, Elinor Accampo, in her study on the nineteenth century decline of birth-rates in France, seeks to reverse 'the traditional questions that demographers seek to answer. Rather than enquire why and how the French stopped having children, it examines the impact of the long-term decline on certain aspects of French political culture, and what the French thought about birth control.' (Accampo 2003: 238). Feminist interventions in demography too have attempted to shift emphasis from the 'big picture' of broad demographic changes to the local and the micro contexts of change, to generate non-linear accounts of change which take conflict, resistance, and culture seriously (Greenhalgh and Li 1995; McDaniel 1996; Bledsoe et al. 1997; Kaler 2000) The present work actively draws upon the sensitivity to power in such interdisciplinary effort to pose the question of fertility change afresh, and is primarily concerned with contextualizing the popularization of birth control in Kerala within emergent regimes of power.

A fourth set of studies that form an important context of this work has been the output of feminist scholars in the 1990s who, troubled by questions similar to mine, investigated the so-called 'gender paradox' of the Kerala Model.[8] One of the earliest critical feminist questions regarding the success of family planning in Kerala was raised by one of Kerala's first feminist social scientists, K. Saradamoni, in a footnote to her article on women, reproduction, and work in Tamil Nadu and Kerala, published in the early 1990s. She asked:

> One hears a lot about the success stories about family planning in Kerala. Generally they are being given out as the achievements of the implementing authority. We have to see this from the point of view of the people, particularly women, who agree to accept them. What are their expectations? Are they being satisfied? What is the regional variation in this? (Saradamoni 1992: 167)

In the past decade feminist historians and social scientists have critically questioned Kerala's interconnected 'golden ages' of community reform and social development to point out that these were also times in which new forms of patriarchal power emerged and were institutionalized here. In the light of this new work, the twentieth century 'liberation' of women in Malayali society has been substantially qualified. Besides, a growing body of critical feminist historical writings has highlighted the reduction of the history of birth control in India to one of fertility control in the demographic literature (for instance, Anandhi 1998). In particular, these writings reveal, (a) how the justification of birth control in terms of women's right to control their bodies was viewed with suspicion; (b) how, by comparison, other endorsements continued to treat female bodies as reproductive (Ramusack 1989; Ahluwalia 2001); and (3) how the discussion of contraception has stayed within the terms of the nation's agenda, even when contraception for the élite has often moved away from narrow population-management goals (John 1998). Another set of writings relevant to this work train a critical eye on global and state policy in reproductive health, reproductive health care, and health provisioning in India (Ravindran 1993; Qadeer 1998; Rao 2004).

Equally important, too, are the debates among feminists on the significance of birth control in the struggle against patriarchy. Feminist observers have reminded us that in the south, women have been made to carry most of the burden of reproduction, and almost by extension, of birth control (Correa and Reichman 1994; Wilson 1994; Lingam 1994). This literature has called attention to the neglect of needs voiced by the women's movement and the instrumentalist use of women's autonomy in population management rhetoric. It engages with and draws upon the critiques of reproductive technology developed by feminists in the developed world. Feminist writings on reproductive technology and control, however, have moved away from both the unequivocal identification of birth control technology as tools of relentless male control over women's reproductive capacities (for instance, as in Corea 1985). Historical and sociological studies have asserted that women are not merely victims of reproductive–technological manipulation, but have sometimes actually demanded them, though the demands have not always been met by the technologies made available (Gordon 1976; Lewis 1980; Petchesky 1985). Nevertheless, within contemporary feminist debates, this does not lead directly to the simple endorsement of the demand for women's bodily autonomy. Recent critical feminist reflections on contraception and personal autonomy have problematized the very concept of autonomy as deriving from the patriarchal notion of 'ownership' (Poovey 1992; Petchesky 1990; Obermeyer 1994). It has also been pointed out that contemporary rhetoric of fertility control reduces women's autonomy to willed pregnancy, and projects this as an absolute necessity that women are obliged to preserve (Ruhl 2002). The very idea that bodily processes ought to be under the control of a rational subject has been used to sanction legislation aimed at scrutinizing the behaviour of pregnant women and mothers in the interests of foetal protection (Daniels 1993). These reflections seem to indicate that no conveniently uncomplicated resolution seems to be in sight within feminist thinking on the topic. This further compounds the task of developing a gender-sensitive perspective on reorienting contraception as a relevant and enabling tool. This may require careful contextual analysis, with an inbuilt wariness towards one-size-fits-all solutions. In any event, feminists interested in birth control have had quite an uneasy relation with the population control lobby (Smyth 1998; Ortiz-Ortega and Helzner 2003). As Nancy Folbre remarks, 'When feminists propose political innovations that help families "catch up" with the effects of social change, to adapt to such trends as fertility decline, they enjoy a certain popularity. But when feminists press beyond "adaptive" prescriptions to suggest ways in which women might actively speed up the transformation of family life, they meet with substantial resistance.' (Folbre 1998: 134).

Through the Literature

I should begin with the existing literature on demographic change and social development in Kerala. This is to distinguish broadly the major methodological orientations in the literature, and the specific kinds of institutions they feed. That will serve to demarcate the different perspectives in the field and establish the claim that this work produces alternative knowledge in the field.

A prominent strand in the study of demographic issues and social engineering in Kerala is wedded to a deductivist theoretical orientation, and draws upon empiricist research methodology. Institutionally, this is linked to the needs of the state and associated agencies to implement a population policy. The areas from which such knowledge has been produced vary from research carried out to aid the family planning programme in the 1950s (Myrdal 1968: 2151–64), to the output of population research centres set up in the states (Rao and Raju 1997). Sharing fully the spirit and letter of what Szreter identifies as characteristic of the reigning notion of 'the scientific study' of population issues (Szreter 1993), in greater or lesser measure, this knowledge too assumes that the initial conditions defining the subject of study can be specified in advance. A methodology that elucidates the mutual cause and effect relationships among the elements in the closed system automatically follows, which offers not just explanation, but also prediction. Producing quantifiable and predictive information, this 'useful' knowledge eminently suits the purpose of planners and policy-makers. Indeed, a sizeable share of such efforts focused upon micro-sites, more or less 'closed systems' such as a family planning camp (Nair and Nair 1978: 147–86) or a limited population such as 'workers in estates and factories' (Nair and Nair 1978: 223–95). Largely un-self-reflexive, it was shaped by the assumptions of state-centric developmentalism and permitted the instrumentalist use of radical slogans (such as freedom from patriarchy). A critical historical perspective, as also the political investment in providing larger choices for individuals, remains alien to this strand. In Kerala, the studies conducted by the demographic research centre were strongly marked by this orientation (Kurup and Mathen 1966; Kurup et al. 1978; Nair and Nair 1978; Varghese 1983).

Another equally or more conspicuous strand is the literature on demographic issues produced within research institutions not directly wedded to the state's need for information, oriented towards initiating a richer understanding of long-term processes in demographic change. Much of this has fed academic as well as the policy debates on development at various levels: local, national, and global. In the context of Kerala, a good example is that of the discussion around the specific processes that caused birth-rates to fall in the twentieth century. Much of the work around these may be broadly characterized as 'structuralist' in orientation, in the sense that it emphasizes the structural changes in the economy, state, and society in explaining broad patterns of social change (Nair 1974; Krishnan 1976; Ratcliffe 1978). Nonetheless 'people' and their ability to exert pressure on the state did emerge as an important element in this literature (Caldwell 1986), without however, damaging its structuralist orientation. We still have the assumption of society as a 'closed system' but the constitutive elements are described at a higher level of complexity. Though it largely hovers within the vision of state-centred development, the state's demand for information is not immediate and the state itself becomes another element of the system to be observed. It feeds into the international debate on population and development in a crucial way, with specific and recognizable effects upon development theory and policy-making as 'useful' knowledge, and is in turn influenced by these.

History is often an important presence in this body of work, serving to provide narratives of social change unfolding in linear progression. The interruptions and digressions in these are sometimes acknowledged, but never strongly enough to provoke a rethinking of the linearity of social change. The demographic transition and popular approbation of artificial birth control appear as though they were the telos of the historical process. Elsewhere, this idea has by now been thoroughly dismantled: the historical studies undertaken in the latter half of the twentieth century indicate that the historical record of north-western Europe does not indicate a consistent and precise link between fertility decline and social, economic, and mortality changes (Thornton 2001). Indeed, the influence of 'developmental idealism' originating from north-western Europe, and relayed throughout the world in the twentieth century (Thornton 2001: 461), on family change is now frequently documented in the scholarship.[9]

The implicit legitimation of the state as the active agent of change in some of the above-mentioned work is accompanied by an uncritical endorsement of the discursive and institutional network in and through which people are made subjects of modern political power. However, a simple acknowledgement of people's agency does not explain the shaping of top–down and gender-insensitive systems of learning and health care. Robin Jeffrey's account (2003) which highlights the public demand for contraception (among other things) in the context of competitive politics in mid-twentieth century Kerala, leaves us with the impression that the Malayali people, fired by developmental idealism, chose and demanded contraception—and the state complied. It certainly does not help us understand how contraception as 'family planning' has necessitated the setting up of a non-reciprocal relation of power between providers and seekers of contraception, and unequal relations between husbands and wives, adults and teenagers, and men and women in general.

However, some of the insights of economists and demographers on Kerala's demographic transition do offer crucial entry points for a critical inquiry into the question of gender and power raised above. It has, for example, been proposed that the higher literacy of women in Kerala (and thus higher ages of marriage) may be more a result of male education than female autonomy (Bhat and Rajan 1990; Rajan et al. 1996). Much earlier, T.N. Krishnan made similar observations in his study of Kerala's fertility transition (1976). As will be clear later, some of these leads have been built upon in this book.

Research that seeks to grasp an 'insider's view'—the meaning of concepts that rule the lives of actors and the community—is a third strand not as prolific as the above two, but growing. This effort is significantly different from studies of popular attitudes to family planning undertaken as part of expanding the knowledge base of the state. The latter aims at assessing the prevalence of pro- and anti-attitudes to family planning, seeking explanations for whatever patterns are discerned and suggesting remedial measures. The former converges upon how actors come to recognize family planning as an essential component of their lives. Indeed, the little research in this vein available on Kerala (largely with disciplinary affiliations to anthropology and sociology) has yielded insights that go far beyond those offered by, for example, the KAP surveys. The anthropologist Marion den Uyl records, for instance, the degree to which family planning in the form of sterilization has been perceived as a social necessity in a dalit settlement in a district in Kerala. She also notes how it has become a social norm, and how drastically unequal the access to Family Planning is for men and women (den Uyl 1995: 181–5). Sociologist K.E. Varghese records the solidification of Family Planning as a compulsive social norm in the Kuttanad area (Varghese 1986: 161–70). These observations can form productive starting points in devising broader questions for research. Marion den Uyl, for instance, connects the unqualified success of family planning among women in the dalit colony to the gradual undermining of motherhood, a situation in which motherhood continues to be passionately desired, but one that is increasingly difficult to support from a material point of view (den Uyl 1995). Filippo and Caroline Osella link the widespread demand for female sterilization and the fervently-kept two-child norm to the upwardly-mobile aspirations of people here (Osella and Osella 2000: 145–6). The efforts to gain an insider's understanding must necessarily be coupled with the efforts to trace the unacknowledged and unarticulated socio–economic and cultural transformations shaping the phenomenon studied. Marion den Uyl's work traces the transformation of motherhood among a particular group of Malayalis in the latter decades of the twentieth century. Such micro-studies, while remaining distinct, complement this effort at delineating a broader critical perspective on how the family planning propaganda in Kerala proved appealing to groups from highly varied social, economic, and geographical situations.

Method

As I have stated earlier, this work is part of an on going endeavour to critically engage with the reigning developmentalist common sense about the un-coerced acceptance of family planning in Kerala. To this end, I have largely relied upon historical analysis. Unlike some of the above-mentioned work, I view society as an uneven, historically mutable, multi-layered, conflict-ridden area. Society is an open system, radically indeterminate. Change in society occurs in irreversible sequences of events, and all the initial conditions can never be specified. As observed earlier, history functions within the entrenched knowledge of demographic change in Kerala as teleology. Here, however, it would serve a very different purpose. It would break down rather than bolster commonsensical associations that wear the air of being 'natural'. For instance, historical analysis would work to show that widespread recognition of family planning as an instrument of economic growth amongst the Malayali public was attained not instantly but at a certain politico–economic conjuncture. It would also show that the recognition of 'population' as the root of all collective and individual ills did not automatically create assent for artificial contraception. Alternatively, it would unbind the taken-for-granted association between the small family and the nuclear family in Kerala, seeking to unravel the specific circumstances under which the two came to be viewed as more or less the same. Historical analysis would also serve to unsettle entrenched ways of viewing the role of civil society. It is often assumed that the remarkable spread of community reform movements of the early twentieth century paved the way by spreading 'enlightened consciousness'. Critical feminist historical analysis here however may highlight the degree to which the thoroughly non-reciprocal relationships of power established within community reformisms were reproduced within family planning in the 1960s. Unabashedly instrumentalist use of the rhetoric of 'liberation' was at the heart of the family planning propaganda throughout India. In Kerala, however, the existence of a long precedent of reformism added to its effectiveness. Not all continuities are repudiated outright; it is only that they are not assumed at the outset, as some of the mainstream literature would have it. This account may not be found wanting in continuities, but they may be ones that have hitherto remained relatively unnoticed. Historical analysis, then, serves to construct a critical account of the popularity of state-centric family welfare in Kerala that goes beyond identifying success or lacunae in the implementation process and the institutional set-up (which in itself is quite valuable).

Relying on such a conception of historical analysis, this work eschews large-scale causal explanations and, indeed, substitutes it with the reconstruction of a historical conjuncture. Here the debt to post-structuralist history writing is transparent (Noujain 1986–7). However, it may be stressed that different social groups in Kerala were drawn towards family limitation through artificial birth control in distinct ways, even while within the above-mentioned larger context; the specific contexts and 'initial conditions' of different social groups are of key significance here. Again, it is important to emphasize the distinct temporal dynamics. All sections of the Malayali people eventually came around to view family limitation as beneficial but it should not be assumed straightway that they all travelled at the same pace along the same route. Sustained documentation of all the varied pathways cannot be replaced with sweeping generalizations or confined to any single work.

I do not, however, undertake such a project of documentation, which would be much larger than any single work. This would call for extensive ethnographic field research, which I have not conducted. This also underlines for some of the limitations of this work: the more-or-less complete reliance on textual sources limits one's investigation of the resistance to and subversions of the state's project. A few instances, which arise in the debates, are mentioned, and indeed, they cry out for a fuller investigation and the use of a more complex set of methodological tools. While this work falls largely within the critical feminist fertility studies approach which looks at reproduction and sexuality as emergent local phenomenon, which are areas of conflict and struggle between groups (Hammel 1990; Greenhalgh and Li 1995), it does fall short of pursuing feminist methodological interventions in the field (McDaniel 1996) to the fullest. The question of how the new technology of fertility control interacted with social relations and how people appropriated them in specific contexts is raised briefly but not followed through with substantial ethnographic fieldwork.

Textual analysis, which is not of social scientific provenance, but now effectively adapted to the purposes of critical social research (Shapiro 1984), is a major tool employed in this work. The idea of the 'text' is a valuable acquisition from literary theory, particularly efficacious in politicizing naturalized, apparently interest-neutral figurations and domains. Displacing both the referent (say, for example, an object 'population') and its intentional consciousness (the subject, the author, the expert, the planner etc.), it places the text at the heart of analysis. The 'text', however, is not seen as a set of symbols that represent objects, but as a set of signs that actively *generate* objects and subjects. There is also the effort to introduce imagery that challenges apparently power-neutral figures. For instance, I would like to recognize the shift from the earlier forms of family to the nuclear family form in twentieth century Malayali society as a process of 'domestication' so that the newer networks of power instituted in and through it become more visible.

I wish to offer below a few broad sketches on three distinct but interrelated ways in which people were interpellated as the subjects of family planning in Malayali society: as self-disciplined and gendered individuals, as responsible householders/homemakers, and as patriotic citizens of the (sub-)nationality of Kerala. In one sense it is committed to careful empirical documentation of the twists and turns of the public discussion on birth control and closely related issues in the period specified. The sources are chiefly drawn from textual material produced in the Malayali public sphere between the 1930s and the 1970s, which include newspaper reports, articles from magazines, public speeches, propaganda material, books, pamphlets, official reports, discussions in legislative bodies, literary writings, and the like. However, central concern is not the accumulation of new 'facts' about the past, but rather to break the self-evidence of these 'facts' and probe the conditions in which they acquire particular kinds of meaning in particular times and spaces. For example, the point is not really to establish that contraception was regarded with suspicion as a threat to social morality at a certain time and among certain groups of people but rather to investigate the conditions that made such an assessment of the significance of contraception possible. Again, the point is not merely to record the shift in which contraception, perceived earlier as dangerously immoral, came to be regarded as an effective safeguard of public morality and domestic harmony, and also to trace the specific conditions for such change. For example, the shift in key notions regarding the nature and social functions of sex and marriage, the emergent forms of power in Malayali society to which the family planning programme could be effectively anchored, and the like.

Through History

The history of welfare in the three political units later united to form the State of Kerala—the British Indian district of Malabar, and the princely states of Cochin (Kochi) and Travancore (Tiruvitamkoor)—was chronologically different. In Travancore, the modern welfare state began taking shape quite early in the nineteenth century, under the tutelage of the colonial power. As early as 1817, Rani Lakshmi Bai of Travancore issued the Royal Rescript stating that the cost of the general education of the people was to be borne by the state, so that 'by diffusion of education they might become better subjects and public servants, and the reputation of the state might be enhanced thereby' (Ramachandran 2000: 102–3). Inaugurating the new Civil Hospital in Thiruvananthapuram in 1865, the Maharajah of Travancore translated Travancore's self-characterization as *Dharma Rajyam* into modern terms, recognizing charity as 'one of the cardinal duties of the state'. 'What can be more real' he asked, 'more substantial charity, than the provision of means for the relief or mitigation of sickness and disease!'[10] Cochin too turned to welfare policies, especially in education and health, from the late nineteenth century. These underwent dramatic expansion between the 1860s and the early 1940s. Malabar, as part of the Madras Presidency, remained much behind both in education and health, and had to wait until after Independence to catch up with Cochin and Travancore.

By the late nineteenth and early twentieth centuries, a class of newly educated élite had begun to make their presence felt in these regions. Several factors worked to ensure a growing demand for modern education. It came to be actively sought with the expansion of activities fuelled by the expansion of state and other institutions in the three regions, and by the integration of Kerala's economy into the capitalist world-system, which accelerated by the late nineteenth century. Missionary work in all those three areas intensified in the nineteenth century, bringing new material, intellectual, and moral resources to challenge the established hierarchies of caste. The late nineteenth century saw the opening up of new 'fields'—legislative, legal, political, and commercial—which required specific skills. Around this period, nascent identities came to be asserted through memorials submitted to the state, such as the Malayali Memorial (1891) and the Ezhava Memorials (1896 and 1900) in Travancore (Jeffrey 2003). The stage was being set for the consolidation of new community identities through the active reformulation of caste groups through community organizations such as the Sree Narayana Dharma Paripalana Yogam, the Nair Service Society, the Nambutiri Yogakshema Sabha, the Sadhujana Paripalana Sangham, and the Araya Samajam. These organizations sought to modernize their respective caste groups, and to actively negotiate with the state about claims over material and cultural resources; they grew at a remarkable pace in the early decades of the twentieth century. The reform of marriage, lineage, and family, and the acquisition of educational and other skills to ensure the inclusion of community members in the newly-opened fields in Malayali modernity, were paramount among their concerns (Awaya 1996; Velayudhan 1999; Kodoth 2001; Arunima 2003). In Travancore, the passing of the Nair Bill in 1925, which allowed individual partition of matrilineal joint family property, signalled the culmination of the long-standing crisis of the Nair matrilineal joint family (Saradamoni 1999). This was followed by legislation that weakened or ended the joint family in other communities too (Jeffery 2003: 43–44). The increasing dissolution of joint families, the economic crises in the wake of the Great Depression, and the consequences of falling of death rates to individual families in the 1920s (Panikar and Soman 1984: 35–6), were all important in provoking public debate around the 'population problem' in the 1930s.

One of the striking features of public life in all three areas in the 1920s and 1930s seems to have been the entry of the first generation of modern-educated women into the public arena, who had begun to be employed in schools, medical institutions, and the government (Devika 2005). These women largely came from the upper castes—Nairs and Syrian Christians—along with others from Ezhava families. Community reformism was peaking, with radical variants of Malayala brahmin reformism coming to the fore (Babu 2001) and the SNDP and NSS entrenching themselves in the emergent political domain. Nationalism peaked in Malabar in the early 1930s, and community-based political opposition to entrenched princely rule heightened in Travancore and Cochin throughout the same decade. These brought to the fore many women activists (Menon 1972). Along with nationalism, community reform efforts, heightened community politics in Travancore and Cochin, and early socialist and trade union assertions, the 1930s also saw the articulation of demands made upon the government on behalf of 'women' as a group, for job reservations, representation in political bodies, and the like. This was however resented by almost all the elements in the political spectrum, and finally overshadowed by the immense growth of communist influence in the late 1930s and '40s. The elitist orientation of these early feminist intellectuals, too, aided their speedy dismissal.

Also, by the 1930s, 'development' had arrived in Travancore. The Marthandam Project, guided by Spencer Hatch, director of Rural Demonstration and Training in Travancore, aimed at improving the lives of rural people by enhancing their incomes through better production techniques and marketting channels (Hatch 1932). The representatives of the Rockfeller Foundation, invited to Travancore to help in organizing a public health department on modern lines, on arrival, found the state 'with its high rates of literacy, wide circulation of newspapers, network of hospitals and trained medical personnel, as most suited for public health work' (Kabir 2003: 12). In ten years, the Foundation did considerable work on hookworm infestation and epidemics such as malaria and filariasis, and opened institutions such as the Neyyattinkara Health Unit near Thiruvananthapuram (Kabir 2003). Public health education on maternal and child health had also begun by the late 1930s in Travancore, and the medium of instruction ranged from newspaper articles to film shows on the subject (Pillai [1940] 1996: 810–11). The situation of course was vastly different in Malabar, as a province of the Madras Presidency: the death rate in Malabar was double that of those in Travancore and Cochin in the mid-'50s (Jeffrey 2003: 191). Here, however, a different form of health activism was taking shape. During the massive cholera epidemic of the early 1940s, the communists organized anti-cholera teams that went from house to house giving advice on preventive measures (Jeffrey 2003: 191). Thus, early in the decades of interest, both the public health machinery as well as the 'citizens' initiative', both of which would be actively drawn upon later for the family planning popularization, were already crystallizing here.

The rise of socialist and communist politics in the 1930s and its remarkable spread in the 1940s ensured the hegemony of leftist ideas in the Malayali cultural sphere in the decades of interest here. In the 1950s, for instance, the leftists won considerable mileage, often across political affiliations, with their uncompromising insistence on the need to unite the three Malayalam-speaking areas of Travancore, Cochin, and Malabar into the state of Kerala (*Aikyakeralam*) (Devika 2004)). This however did not mean the end of community politics. The communists were ranged against highly organized community interests and Congress nationalists, who were not reduced to passivity (Mammen 1981) Indeed, this is a period of striking political turbulence—marked by the first communist ministry (1957–9)—even though leftist intellectuals were able to set the terms of most debates. Indeed, as many others have noted, the period saw significantly strong welfarist and anti-poverty measures initiated by the state, among which the family planning programme is counted as significant. The 1960s saw the decline of the Nehruvian promises of regional development, and distress in the backdrop of war, drought, and the subsequent food crisis—and this precipitated intense agitation in the Malayali public sphere. Both these were crucial in the successful projection of family planning as a panacea for Malayali ills, as we shall see.

The Arguments, Summarized

The three chapters that follow work through the mass of written materials that accumulated around birth control as a topic of public interest in these times. The first of these traces the shift in the attitude towards birth control evident in public debates on the issue, from the 1930s to the early 1970s. Frequently opposed in the 1930s as entirely inimical to individual self-disciplining—a goal set for all individuals aspiring to be 'modern' by all forms of reformism—artificial contraception came to be seen in entirely different terms by the 1960s. Intervening between these decades were a range of cultural and social transformations that simply cannot be encapsulated under such cliched formulations as the 'expansion of enlightened consciousness'. They included significant changes in the way sex and sexual desire came to be understood, and in conceptions of marriage and conjugality that accompanied the massive restructuring of marriage, family and kin ties in the twentieth century. The calcification of modern forms of 're-formist' patriarchy, in which modernized men claim the authority to design and oversee the implementation of 'women's liberation', and the entrenchment of the new élitism of modern scientific knowledge that marginalized all other ways of knowing, were important developments that mediated these changes. The debate that unfolded in the subsequent decades often set itself the task of reconciling artificial contraception to the self-disciplining endeavours of individuals. Indeed, by the 1960s, this seemed to have been successfully accomplished, through the revisioning of sex, sexual desire, and conjugality. Simultaneously, the 'missionary mode of subject-production' which operated through what Michel Foucault calls the modern 'pastoral', was harnessed as the most efficient means of securing social government. The reference, of course, is to the newer, hither-worldly version of pastoral power, which retains the sacrificial, individualizing, lifelong qualities of the earlier mode, and continues to emphasize the individual conscience as the seat of self-regulation of society.

The second chapter attempts to trace the shaping of certain life-options emergent in Malayali modernity that increasingly mobilized the desire of ever-greater sections of Malayali society, and directed them towards the small family norm. I argue that we need to follow the process of 'domestication' to which the Malayalis seem to have been subjected in this period at much greater length and detail than in this work. By 'domestication' I mean a process by which the larger measure of individual energies and interests have been directed into the interiors of the home and the family, especially into the 'crafting' of children. Starting from around mid-nineteenth century, the entire notion of parental responsibility came to be radically gendered and defined in such a way as to permit the state to 'access' the family. The agencies of the modern father/householder and modern mother/homemaker were constructed in such a way that the state could make a direct appeal to them on behalf of the nation, bypassing all other collective interests that exist in between, such as those of the community or the locality. The gradual consolidation of a notion of family subsistence as involving the balancing of scarce means and burgeoning wants was another crucial notion that waxed strong during this period, at least for some groups. This chapter also takes up the question why other powerful social processes, in which numbers remained quite crucial that were contemporary, such as the prevalence of community politics and the waxing of the (sub-) national identity of Malayalis as natives of Kerala, seemed entirely compatible with the call for a reduction in numbers.

The third chapter focuses on how artificial contraception is finally endorsed as a measure of relevance to society as a whole, as a valuable support for the state's economic growth, linked to the transformation of local society into one capable of efficient utilization of economic resources. Severe anxieties about sub-national identity and delayed economic take-off formed a crucial backdrop against which family planning came to be cogently presented as a practical instrument of economic development. By the early 1950s, 'population' was already identified as the major pathogen behind Kerala's economic ills, through, and in many, separate discussion-contexts. I examine here three distinct contexts: (a) around the food deficit, that began to appear with increasing integration into the world economy, (b) around rising unemployment, (c) around the 'beggar problem' in the wake of the near-famine conditions during the Second World War. Artificial contraception did not really figure high on the list of remedies proposed. They included intensified agricultural growth, industrialization, and migration, and these solutions were often advanced more forcefully than artificial contraception. However, by the late 1950s, political and economic conditions seemed to be shaping up in such a way that the former three seemed to be more and more unavailable. This endowed family planning with a significance beyond being an instrument of individual sexual self-discipline or family well being. Also, a broad consensus on the utility of Family Planning (henceforth, FP) as beneficial for society in general, at least in the long run, needed to be generated in the Malayali public for it to thrive. This was without a doubt an essential condition for the government's assumption of the role of the primary provider of FP services in Kerala in a dynamic and commanding sense. It is argued that the legitimation of FP as an important economic solution was also important in ensuring that developmentalism in Kerala had a longer lease of life than elsewhere in India.

The three chapters that form the core of this work seek to open new avenues to explore and new questions to investigate; they do not pretend to offer final answers. The fervent hope is that these will do the work of a rock flung into stagnant waters – while the inertness is pierced by vigorous ripples, I am prepared to accept that the rock itself may disappear beneath the waters. We probably need more of such misshapen and discomfiting rocks and less of (intellectual) monuments that inspire awed silence.

Notes

1 For a fuller discussion on the 'Kerala Model', see G. Parayil (ed.), *Kerala: The Development Experience*, London and New York, Zed Books, 2000; Robin Jeffrey *Politics, Women and Well-being: How Kerala became a 'Model'*, New Delhi, Oxford University Press, 2003.

2 Organized by the District Collector of Ernakulam, S.S. Krishnakumar, in December 1970, in which 15,000 people were sterilized. See Mohan Rao, *From Population Control to Reproductive Health: Malthusian Arithmetic*, New Delhi, Sage Publications, 2004, 39–40.

3 It is yet another matter, of course, that the quality of health care focused on women in Kerala leaves much to be desired. Observing a laproscopic sterilization camp in Kerala in 1993, researchers found that women were not even aware of the minimum standard of care that was due to them, and that their dignity as individuals was scarcely considered by service providers. See Mala Ramanathan et al., 'Quality of Care in Laproscopic Sterilisation Camps: Observations from Kerala, India', *Reproductive Health Matters* 3, 6, 1995, 84–93. Nor is the access to sterilization always equal. Marion den Uyl, working in a dalit colony in Kerala, notes that while family planning workers expected women to obtain written permission from their husbands, men could opt for sterilization on their own. M. den Uyl, *Invisible Barriers: Gender, Caste and Kinship in a Southern Indian Village*, Utrecht, International Books, 1995, 181.

4 It appears that at least in the 1960s family planning technocrats and bureaucrats were no less advocates of covert coercion. It was the lack of unanimity in political society that stalled the institution of indirect coercion. Dr C.O. Karunakaran, foremost among Kerala's crusading FP doctors, noted with disappointment in 1968 that 'It was Kerala's Family Planning Board and Seminars which first argued in favour of indirect coercive measures. It was also the Government of Kerala that limited maternity leave to three months first, during the Advisor's period. After that, though other States have adopted more efficient

measures, Kerala has not moved a foot forward. The United Front has not been united in this matter...' C.O. Karunakaran, 'Kudumbasamvidhanam Avideyum Ivideyum' (Family Planning There and Here), *Kerala Kaumudi*, 18 May 1968, 2.

[5] While 1545 vasectomies were conducted in Kerala in 2000–1, 149,498 tubectomies were done; in 1999–2000, the corresponding figures were 653 and 153,515. See the state-wise urban and rural break-up of vasectomies, tubectomies, and total sterilizations, 1999–2001 and 2000–1 in Go I 2003: Tables C3.2 and C3.3. An evaluation of the family welfare programme in Kerala carried out in 1992 points out that since 1974, tubectomies have accounted for about 98.8 per cent of total sterilizations. M. Nessimunnissa Beevi, 'An Evaluation of Family Welfare Programme in Kerala, India', in G.N. Rao (ed.) *Family Planning: The Afro-Asian Scenarios*, Research Monograph Series Vol. 5. Thiruvananthapuram, Centre for Development Studies, 1999, 235.

[6] Not that this has gone entirely unnoticed, though such instances still seem very rare. See for instance, Frank Furedi, *Population and Development: A Critical Introduction*. Oxford, Polity Press, 1997, 134–5.

[7] The editors of a recent special issue of the *Journal of Interdisciplinary History* advocate an approach that 'joins the quantitative strengths of demographic history with the interpretive power of cultural and oral history. The former can pinpoint when, where, and among whom significant changes in family formation occurred, but texts and testimonies are indispensable for a more complete understanding of why those changes occurred and what they meant to the groups and communities involved ... [birth controllers] have arrived at their current practices through an enormous variety of pathways'. S. Szreter, R.A. Nye and F. van Poppel, 'Fertility and Contraception during the Demographic Transition: Quantitative and Qualitative Approaches', *Journal of Interdisciplinary History* 34, 2, 2003, 154.

[8] Anna Lindberg, *Experience and Identity: A Historical Account of Class, Caste and Gender among the Cashew Workers of Kerala, 1930–2000*, Lund, Department of History, University of Lund, 2001; Monica Erwer, *Challenging the Gender Paradox: Women's Collective Agency in the Transformation of Kerala Politics*. Goteborg, Department of Peace and Development Studies, Goteborg University, 2003; J. Devika, *En-Gendering Individuals: The Language of Re-forming in Early 20th Century Keralam*, Hyderabad, Orient Longman, 2007. Praveena Kodoth and Mridul Eapen, 'Looking Beyond Gender Parities: Gender Inequities of Some Dimensions of Well-Being in Kerala', *Economic and Political Weekly*, 40, 30, 2005, 3278–86; Sharmila Sreekumar, 'Scripting Lives: Narratives by Dominant Women in a Southern State', Ph.D. thesis submitted to Hyderabad Central University, 2001. See also F. Osella and C. Osella, *Social Mobility in Kerala: Modernity and Identity in Conflict*, London, Pluto Press, 2001 for not explicitly critical but certainly 'post-Kerala Model' analysis of social life in contemporary Kerala.

[9] The intellectual history of demography as a social science discipline has thrown

interesting insights on the very idea of 'demographic transition'. It has been historicized and critiqued to show that it was intimately bound to the ever-greater entrenchment of policy considerations within demography. (D.Hodgson, 'Demography as a Social Science and Policy Science', *Population and Development Review* 9, 1, 1983, 1–34). C.S. Szreter has also pointed out that 'the principal virtue and function of the idea of demographic transition has always been in providing a graphic metaphor that summarily describes, and predicts, a long-term overall emergent pattern of change.... [but] a summary description of this metaphorical sort offers no necessary assistance of insight into the causal explanation of how such change occurred or occurs in any particular case. Unless an implicit teleology is subscribed to, it is simply an act of faith to base empirical and historical researches on its premises.' C.S. Szreter, 'The Idea of Demographic Transition and the Study of Fertility Change: A Critical Intellectual History', *Population and Development Review* 19, 4, 1993, 692. For an argument that traces the links between demographic transition theory and colonial demography, see Karl Ittman, 'Demography as Policy Science in the British Empire, 1918–1969', *Journal of Policy History* 15, 4, 2003, 417–48.

10 Speech, reported in *Travancore Administration Report*, 1865–66, 61.

1

Sexual Discipline, 'Liberation' and Family Planning

'Modern against Progress?'

Speaking in the Cochin Legislative Council in 1934, a Member, C.O. Ouseph, opposed a resolution that demanded the Cochin government's support for birth-control clinics in these terms:

> Some, who want to have the enjoyment of actions, want to avoid the obligations of it. Is it not immoral? You want your passions to be satisfied and yet are not ready to bear the resultant burdens.... You are given the power to control yourself. Do you want to remain a man or unman yourself? The result of this resolution is an acceptance of defeat, an admission that the human will cannot control human nature. That, Sir, is dangerously immoral and contributes to continued slavery. [*Proceedings of the Cochin Legislative Council* 1934: 63.]

The late 1920s and 30s saw the peaking of social reformism among the Malayalis. Reformist Malayali intellectuals of the late nineteenth and early twentieth centuries had shown, early enough, an obsession with initiating a 'selection process', or a 'sifting', through which they hoped to create the 'ideal mix' of 'tradition' and 'modernity' best suited to local society. C.O. Ouseph participated in precisely such selection through his critique of artificial contraception. By the late 1920s and early 1930s, the twin thrust of the reformist critique—the critique of the indigenous order, and engagement with much that arrived here marked as 'modern'—had reached unprecedented levels of intensity. An intense period of social change had already gone by. Many indigenous systems and institutions were beginning to crumble at its onslaught. Added to these were the emergent stresses and strains—the effects of Kerala's integration into the world-capitalist economy, the fallouts of the abolition of indigenous joint family forms, the anxieties engendered by new lifestyles and possibilities for consumption.

Pertinent to my inquiry is the fact that commercialized agriculture, the spread of education, and community reformisms in the late nineteenth and early twentieth centuries had ignited, to some extent and degree, what Arland Thornton calls 'developmental idealism' (Thornton 2001), especially in Travancore and Cochin (Tharakan 1992).[1] Of the four propositions that Thornton finds typical of developmental idealism as a global discourse, three were already familiar presences amongst the expanding Malayali public of the late 1920s, with variations in emphases. Briefly stated, the three propositions, in the Malayali context, appeared thus: (a) that modern society—society characterized by technologically sophisticated means of production, capable of high degrees of wealth-creation, institutions that relied on non-coercive forms of control, and populated by industrious, reasonable and skilled individuals—was good and desirable. (b) That the modern family—cast in the model of the north-west European nuclear family model with its attendant values—was both naturally/divinely prescribed and culturally/economically desirable. (c) That the modern family, properly nurtured, would act as a transforming force, erasing indigenous ideas, practices, and finally institutions, and affirming the values of modern society.

The fourth of Thornton's propositions—that individuals are free and equal and social relations are based on consent—appeared here with a number of qualifications. In other words, like elsewhere in India, participants in public discussions here too agreed upon the need for 'freedom' and 'equality', but worried about the implications of welcoming 'Western freedom', or 'Western ideas of equality'. Right from the early twentieth century, there were efforts to define it quite tightly. The modern notion of 'freedom', for instance, was translated as *swatantryam*, or 'self-means for survival', and carefully distinguished from *tantonnittam*—'doing-as-you-please' (Devika 2006).[2] 'Equality', again, was carefully qualified through the gradual building up of new hierarchies and fresh boundaries defined by gender, education, and employment, which not so much displaced earlier forms, as transformed or overlaid them. The modern-educated new élite in Kerala, which was shaped through a partial breach of the earlier caste-based 'order of difference by birth', which rapidly attained a hegemonic position in society in mid twentieth century, rested precisely upon these new hierarchies and boundaries.[3]

This peculiar configuration of developmental idealism was to prove decisive in shaping the debates around artificial contraception here: few other practices that bore the label of the 'modern' aroused so much anxiety at the very outset.[4] The fears that it aroused were manifold, but they certainly cannot be readily assigned to categories like 'orthodox–traditional objections', or 'superstitious fears'. The section that follows roughly outlines these. To put it very briefly, it was feared that artificial contraception would undermine the project of shaping sexually disciplined modern individuals, so highly cherished by social reformers, undo the fundamental physiological conditions necessary for the actualization of ideal complementarity between the genders, and thus gnaw at the very base of the much-desired institution of the modern family. Indeed, if the attainment of 'progress' (the developmental paradigm within which developmental idealism makes sense) was contingent upon the attainment of modern society and family, then this appeared to be a practice destructive of both. Nothing short, then, of a case of 'modern against progress'.

However, if one were to cut suddenly to the 1960s, a dramatic change would be evident. In 1934, a humour-magazine, *Rasikan* had poked fun at A. Balakrishna Pillai, a leading modernist intellectual and fervent advocate of artificial birth control in these terms:

> In the end, the government must seek to promote understanding about the excess number of children by beginning a study-centre in every taluk,

> which would inquire about and understand procreation, its timing, number, practice and place. If necessary, the editor of *Kesari*, Balakrishna Pillai B.A.B.L. will supervise and control such schools.[5]

In the late 1960s this would have no longer appeared a joke. In the vigorous campaigns for family planning, all the earlier associations made by its critics were reversed. Now, artificial birth control was no longer associated with sexual profligacy but with sexual discipline, concern about procreation and socialization of the young, and with abstentious living; with the perpetuation of modern domestic life and not its abrogation; with procreative, not pleasure-seeking female sexuality. Indeed, artificial birth control did not even appear to be a travesty of nature, but rather an instrument that aided individuals to get in tune with nature within themselves. In a span of around thirty years, a remarkable transformation appeared to have occurred in the understanding of artificial contraception, at least among the Malayali new élite.

How do we make sense of this change? The following section tries to present the major arguments advanced against birth control in the early decades of the twentieth century. I then go on to examine the transformations undergone by the key concepts that underpinned the entire debate around marriage, sexuality, family, and contraception in order to make sense of the shift from suspicion to acceptance. I pursue the vicissitudes of the transformation of associations in the discourse on love (*premam*) and lust (*kamam*), the functions of modern conjugality and the forces sustaining it, and the balance of forces within the modern nuclear family. These, I claim, were vital in assuring public acceptance of artificial birth control as a viable, indeed, necessary solution to a variety of ills perceived to be plaguing mid-twentieth century Malayali society.

While the FP propaganda used the new cultural-ideological space that was being shaped to its advantage, its design aided the intensive spread of the cultural and social values of the modern educated élite. It stayed well within that local variant of Victorian morality that characterized the new élite. Emergent and growing since the nineteenth century, this sexual morality relied upon self-disciplining as the major mode of regulating desire, on heterosexuality as the major mode of defining sexual desire and practice, and on patriarchy as the major power organizing relations between the sexes. The institution that was to house it was undoubtedly the modern nuclear family—provided for chiefly by the father, and supervised internally by the mother. In turn, this institution was to be maintained through adherence to the former. Indeed, FP propaganda was also instrumental in carrying such moral norms to a number of groups hitherto relatively isolated. Alongside this, it assiduously evoked the élitism of knowledge—between the educated élite and the 'masses', between contraceptive providers and users.

The last section examines these aspects. It seeks to illustrate how the inherent 'progressiveness' attributed to the FP Programme (FPP from now) both rested upon and furthered the emergent forms of power in modern Malayali society that defined and guided its modernization. Particularly prominent is modern patriarchy (largely reliant on persuasion, and less on direct coercion) in which (modern educated) men design and oversee the process of 'women's liberation'. Equally important are the new élitism of modern knowledge, and the 'passivizing' power of reformist 'uplifting' which authorizes non-reciprocal relations of power between the subject of reform and the objects to be reformed.

Discipline vs. Government?

The early arguments advanced against artificial birth-control often reflected anxieties about realizing the ideal modern self that had begun to be upheld against the older socio–economic and cultural orders ever since the late nineteenth century in Malayali society. From these early times, the project of modern self-building was portrayed as crucially dependent on a high degree of self-disciplining, particularly expressed in sexual self-restraint. This capacity for regulation of the self was seen to be the mark of its 'freedom' (*swatantryam*) and the condition of its integration into modern institutions (Devika 2007).

From the 1930s onwards, i.e. around the period when artificial birth-control came to be actively discussed in the Malayali public sphere, to the late 1950s at least, we find much writing that expresses deep suspicion of artificial contraception as fundamentally incompatible with the project of modern self-building. The idea that vigorous sexual desire was pathological, the conviction that sexual self-control was central to self-building, and the fear that artificial birth-control would open up a Pandora's Box, leading to sexual chaos, were inevitably voiced in such writing. In contrast, natural birth control was hailed as ideal for the sexually-disciplined subject capable of disciplined labour and procreation.[6] These arguments continued to appear sporadically even in the heyday of FP, the 1960s. Undoubtedly, the most vigorous proponents of such arguments were the Catholic publicists (a powerful presence in all public arenas in Kerala); however, the opposition was by no means limited to the Catholic Church alone.[7] The sharp distinction perceived between 'natural' and 'artificial' forms of birth control highlights the degree to which the project of self-regulation had been naturalized. The fact that 'natural' means of birth control were by no means 'natural' as they clearly presupposed the rigorous cultural training of the mind and body was not considered at all. Thus Paul Mampilli, a member of the Cochin Legislative Council in the 1930s, argued during a discussion on the resolution on birth control clinics introduced by the rationalist reformer Sahodaran K. Ayappan that if birth-control was to be attained, it was to be only through staying within the project of 'the control of the mind, by the exercise of will-power' (*Proceedings of the Cochin Legislative Council* 1934: 80). Indeed, for such persons, artificial contraception would be utterly superfluous. At the same time, making it available to the vast majority who had not attained sexual self-control seemed dangerously threatening to the project of modern self-building itself—any sign that they sought or practised it would be already evidence for their deviation from this project.

Later opponents of artificial birth control drew out other objections that followed from such arguments. The Health Survey and Development Committee established in 1943 (the Bhore Committee) to provide a national blueprint for the development of health services in India had in 1946 supported artificial birth control, advancing reasons amply laced with eugenic concerns (quoted in Rao 2004: 24–5). In Kerala, doubts were still strong in many quarters. In a similar discussion on a resolution demanding state support for family planning in the legislative assembly of the unified state of Travancore–Cochin in 1951, A.J. John, the finance minister, remarked that introducing artificial contraception among people who did not even know 'the rudiments of self-control and health care' would invite health hazards, besides stirring up uncontrolled and excessive sexual activity (*Proceedings of the Travancore-Cochin Legislative Assembly* 1952: 1608). For such people, it seemed, the only barrier to the unregulated pursuit of carnal pleasures was the social stigma attached to illegitimate births. Artificial control now seemed to offer them the possibility of evading this censor, thus removing the external controls upon those who in the first place had no internalized controls. This, then, would be a formidable threat to the actualization of a disciplined sexual order yoked to efficient production of wealth and procreation. It can hardly be forgotten that sexual discipline was accepted to be absolutely crucial to the shaping of a modern community in almost every version of community reformism that has appeared in Malayali society (Devika 2007). Not everything issuing out of the West, it was often commented, would help modernity incarnate in Malayali society. Artificial birth control was identified by its critics as a force capable of such 'abortive' effect. As C.O. Ouseph put it (in the opening quotion of this chapter), it seemed to perpetuate 'slavery', which was certainly pre-modern. In a situation in which strong and well-disciplined internalities were ill-formed in subjects, it seemed against the interest of social governance geared to the purpose of accelerating material production, that external constraints be removed.[8] It may, however be noted that this 'regulation by nature' was not read as a rival or threat to the regulatory efforts of social institutions but rather as a support; even the sole support. The parallel between the two was well-illustrated by the well-known humourist of this period, P.K. Rajaraja Varma when he pictured nature as a 'government' extracting a tax from its subjects for the pleasure of sex. Artificial birth control is seen as a means of avoiding this tax; people could now enjoy themselves without 'paying' (Varma 1948: 31).

A second set of related criticisms stemmed from the suspicion that artificial birth control would adversely affect the 'gender contract' that was to be ideally established between man and woman within the modern home. Ever since the nineteenth century a great deal of writing had accumulated around the theme of 'natural' capacities of men and women, which supposedly made them fit to inhabit different social domains, the public and the domestic. One of the major burdens of early twentieth century social reformism in Kerala was to institute such a partitioning of the world in a society in which such distinctions were definitely blurred and fluid. This 'contract' was seen to enable a complementary exchange between men and women for mutual benefit so that the realms of production and procreation would be at once separated and mutually linked, energizing each other (Devika 1999). The seriousness with which this was perceived is hardly surprising, given the fact that the establishment of complementarity between the sexes was considered to be of central importance in the project of forging the modern collectivity, be it the modern church, community, nation, or family. It was feared that artificial birth control would make women 'manly': women would then no longer prefer their proper domain, the modern home, but hanker after 'manly' callings. This would disrupt the complementarity of the sexes and thus affect the mutual energizing of procreation and production. Even those who were sufficiently convinced that womanly capacities had ample application in the public domain and not in the domestic domain alone—such as many of the first generation feminists in Kerala (Devika 2005)—were suspicious of the effects of artificial contraception. Speaking at a meeting of the Neyyattinkara Town Women's Association in 1935, Mrs Malloor Govinda Pillai, a prominent social worker and philanthropist of Travancore, sharply attacked artificial contraception as actually disadvantaging women by prompting them to abandon their socially prestigious role of mother. While unambiguously supporting paid employment and economic independence for women, she opposed artificial birth control as bad strategy, upsetting both body and mind. Along with this was expressed support for natural birth control, recommended to women who could not afford to have children (quoted in Panikker 1954: xxxi–xxxiii). Other critics were harsher; identifying users of artificial contraception as parasitic, sickly, immoral, and pleasure-seeking women who sought artificial birth control, desiring an illegitimate gender-crossing. *Aryakeralam,* criticizing women-supporters of artificial birth control, poured scornful invective on educated women who were supposedly hankering for space in the public domain. They were faulted for being old maids chasing an easy and flighty life, which was then easily read as desiring a reversal of gender roles.[9] Such suspicions were still being voiced in the 1950s by highly educated, articulate, and financially self-reliant Catholic women who favoured only natural birth control. However, it is difficult to characterize these women as somehow bound to conservatism as far as their ideas about gender relations are concerned. We find in their speeches a strong endorsement of associations for women, the entry of women into public life, criticism of governments and political parties for not providing women enough space in the public domain, and calls for alertness on the part of women to national and international affairs.[10] Besides, artificial birth control was feared to impair the reproductive capacities of women's bodies (Kurup 1928; Nair 1932).

Also, artificial birth control was feared to hold the threat of turning the chaste wife into no more than a prostitute; of reducing wives to no more than objects of male sexual desire.[11] The abandonment of sexual passivity by women, whether a consequence of adopting artificial contraception or not, was in general read as a sign of decadence by the progressives and the sceptics alike (Devika 1999). It is no wonder then that many people who supported birth control limited themselves, at least initially, to support for self-control. Anna Chandy, the first Malayali woman to earn a law degree and practice as a lawyer, and a leading feminist of the 1930s in Travancore, initially recommended birth control through self-control (Chandy [1929] 2005), though she later supported artificial birth control actively at the All-India Women's Conference at Thiruvananthapuram in 1934 (Chandy 1935). Much later, Lalitambika Antarjanam, one of the earliest of Malayali women to carve out a space of her own in the nascent institution of modern Malayalam literature, used the debate over the desirability of artificial birth control for women to advance her alternative vision of motherhood that would not participate in the project of fashioning 'hard' Individuals. In her short story *Mulappalinte Manam,* artificial birth control is granted qualified support on condition that what she deemed to be essentially 'womanly'—the ability to transcend the public/private divide and heal the schisms opened up by individualism—should not dry up as a consequence (Antarjanam [1937] 1973). Her explicit support for artificial contraception came much later, in her congratulatory message to the family planning 'festival' at Ernakulam, which had strong overtones of eugenic concerns (*Kerala Kaumudi*, 22 July 1971: 5). In the 1950s, another prominent woman to gain recognition within modern Malayalam literature, K. Saraswati Amma, recommended artificial birth control to the masses (Amma 1958: 47) but reserved birth control through self-disciplining to those women who aspired for an internally oriented, individuated self (Amma 1955: 42). Staunch advocates of women's entry into public life of the 1930s, like R. Easwara Pillai, could go only as far as self-control (Pillai 1936). As for the journals, some like *Kesari* and *Sahodaran* were unwaveringly pro-artificial birth control, while other progressive publications like *Mahila* and *M.N. Nair Masika* published both viewpoints. In "Vanitalokam" (Women's World) column of the *M.N. Nair Masika* of 1936, E.N. Meenakshi Amma wrote thus:

> Our women may run away scared when they hear about contraception. The best way to control the number of births is through self-control. Only that those who find this impossible may seek other means. It is essential that a mother should have children only as far as her health and financial ability allow. Each woman has the responsibility to decide the means by which this may be achieved. [Amma 1936.]

However, in 1938 the same author was arguing against contraception in the same column. Citing a Japanese doctor,

Meenakshi Amma now wrote against the idea that more pregnancies ruined a woman's health: 'In short this Japanese doctor says that more pregnancies are better for the health and longevity of the mother. We know that for women, most illnesses are cured by childbirth.... Woman's physique has been constructed for the purpose of giving birth. Therefore the basis of women's health lies in giving birth.' (Amma 1938). *Mahila*, arguably the leading women's magazine in Malayalam of the early twentieth century, shifted its position in a very short while.[12] In any case, most of the supporters and the opponents of artificial birth control were only too ready to concede that there was a need to reduce numbers in the 'general' interest of society, and that 'natural' birth control was the most desirable and healthy means to this end. Artificial birth control did have its committed proponents—as, for instance, the prominent women's rights advocate, Mrs C. Kuttan Nair (see, Amma 1931; 1991). The point, however, is that modern educated women who agreed otherwise on the advisability of paid employment for women, and their participation in public affairs, did not necessarily agree on the advisability of artificial contraception for women as a means of expanding women's social space.

The third kind of fear about the effects of artificial contraception stemmed directly from the above two: the undermining of the project of modern self-building and the erosion of sexual complementarity seemed to threaten the modern family, and with it, 'civilization' itself. These appear even in the early debates. In 1934, Joseph Pettah raised this point against K. Ayappan's resolution in the Cochin Legislative Council requesting the government's help for those who wished or needed to practice birth control. He argued that large families were better training grounds for children who were to enter a competitive society: 'the children of the large family are much more enterprising, much better fitted to the battle of life than those of the small family ... in the large family, you get a training ground for the development of certain qualities which are essential [to succeed] in the competition of life' (*Proceedings of the Cochin Legislative Council* 1934: 155). More or less the same argument came up in the

Travancore–Cochin legislative assembly in 1951 during the debate on family planning. Speaking on A.P. Udayabhanu's resolution appealing for government support for family planning, A.K. George claimed that large families were more suited to a robust democracy. Citing the example of a twelve-member family, he said: 'They had their own small parliament; they budgeted their own income and so on.' (*Proceedings of the Travancore-Cochin Legislative Assembly* 1952: 1599). The same argument appears in several other texts.[13]

The fears about the destruction of the modern family occupied a prominent place in the Catholic anti-Soviet texts produced in Kerala in the 1940s and 1950s.[14] These often painted a lurid picture of Soviet society as a horde. Soviet people, it was claimed, were being, on the one hand, made to labour like cattle by a tyrannical state; on the other, they were prompted to indulge in mindless pleasure-seeking, which ate into the internal capacity of individuals to resist state tyranny and rationally judge its policies. The destruction of the affective bonds seen to hold together the modern family was identified as the major strategy through which the communist state achieved its overarching powers (for instance, Narikkuzhi 1954: 19). It was further claimed that under such adverse circumstances, the family was supported by little more than a flimsy legality that rendered it highly insecure. The reference was to pre-Stalinist Soviet society, which loosened the restrictions on abortions and contraception; indeed the Stalinist curbs on such access was read as a reaction to the 'damage' caused by this to the fabric of Soviet society (Narikkuzhi 1954: 22). These were very widely circulated—for instance, the text cited above, *Kudumbattinu Nere* (Against the family) had already gone into three editions since 1952, with about 12,000 copies produced (Narikkuzhi 1954, front matter). Communist authors and fellow travellers directly or indirectly fought off such charges. Some claimed that socialism would be a solution to the struggles of low-income groups to support their families. Others argued that Soviet society, and indeed, all socialism, was committed to fostering the procreative family, and that sexual lawlessness was non-existent in the USSR (Menon [1942] 2003: 41–9; Thomas 1948; Damodaran 1952; Nambutiripad 1999; Devadas [1949] 1991: 65–70). Indeed, even those who disagreed with the communists in Kerala in these times were found congratulating them on the strict sexual discipline the party enforced within its ranks, for instance, the non-communist politician of the 1950s, Annie Joseph (Joseph 1954). Several autobiographies of leading communist activists testify to their concern about the need to channel sexual desire into productive channels, and their recognition of the relevance of (a revised version of) modern familial arrangements to secure this (Pisharady 1984; Gopalan 1980; George 1985).

This is not to claim, however, that every single objector to artificial birth control was evenly plagued by such fears as these. Nothwithstanding the unmistakable predominance of the social fears elaborated here, there were some who stressed the economic, rather than the social ailments it could possibly result in, as for instance, the economist P.J. Thomas in the 1930s and '40s, who highlighted the economic advantages of a large population. These will be discussed in the third chapter. Many progressive (and sometimes) left-leaning intellectuals pointed to the fact that the high fecundity of the poor is a rational survival strategy (Kesavadev 1933; Kunhuraman [1938] 2002; Menon 1973: 385). In the debate over A.P. Udayabhanu's resolution seeking support for artificial contraception from the government in the Travancore–Cochin legislative assembly in 1951, communist member E. Gopalakrishna Menon opposed the resolution, and the socialist Daniel Jose assented to it, both carefully qualifying their respective positions. Menon mounted a full-scale attack on the neo-Malthusian roots of the population control drive. He disputed the extension of FP as a national need, while arguing that individuals who decide to avail of contraception should be allowed access (*Proceedings of the Travancore–Cochin Legislative Assembly* 1952: 1601–2). Jose, on the contrary, defended the resolution, but reserved 'self-control' for the elite and clinical methods for the 'labouring masses' with high fecundity (*Proceedings of the Travancore-Cochin Legislative Assembly* 1952: 1591). However, not all of these intellectuals were entirely free of the fears mentioned above. For instance, C.V. Kunhuraman's arguments against artificial birth control were also coloured by eugenics. Birth control advice, he felt, would be put into practice only by people with a certain degree of knowledge. The result would be that 'the number of people with knowledge will go down, and the number of ignorant folk will increase' (Kunhuraman [1938] 2004: 173). The shadow of eugenics in Jose's arguments is obvious. And Gopalakrishna Menon's spirited defence of the individual's right to contraception was somewhat qualified in his entwining of two distinct claims: one, that individuals in Soviet Russia were free to avail of contraception if they so desired, and two, that the population expansion in the 1940s in the USSR was an outcome of the fact that the expanding economy required a larger population. In the socialist utopia that he constructs, the individual, it is implied, cheerfully and almost naturally complies with governmental regulation (*Proceedings of the Travancore–Cochin Legislative Assembly* 1952: 1602–3)—which was precisely what many of his opponents feared.

It is also easily supposed that because a large number of the objectors were Catholics, they were somehow less modern. It may be the case that the Catholic Church advanced such modern objections as the above as a cover up for its conservative adherence to dogma. This however in itself matters little. Whatever be their intentions, it was very clear by the third decade of the twentieth century that in order to frame a convincing case against artificial birth control in the public sphere, it was no longer sufficient to advance religious objections alone. The Catholic Church, even at the height of its anti-communism and anti-rationalism shared the first three propositions of developmental idealism mentioned earlier in this chapter. We have only to see the innumerable articles and speeches endorsing modernization of agriculture, adoption of scientific health-care, industrialization, and other topics that appeared in *Nazrani Deepika*, and in the All-Kerala Catholic Conferences. Religious objections were abundantly voiced within the anti-artificial birth control literature produced by the Catholic Church; but they were certainly not projected as the most important ones. Indeed, it must be stressed that a general agreement that population growth was not to be lightly taken was shaping up between the 1930s and the 1950s; and all agreed that it had to be controlled. The disagreement was over questions of 'how to'.

Indeed, the contours of this debate around artificial contraception are remarkably similar to the debate about birth control in Britain between the late nineteenth and early twentieth centuries, in which both sides pitch their arguments with equal force around the 'consequences for modernity' (Hauck 2003). Perhaps the divergence may not be characterized as one between 'progressives' and 'reactionaries'. The agreements between these sections are noteworthy: both agreed on the necessity to expand governmental regulation of population, expressed in their support for the government's efforts in public health, sanitation, and other areas. Some, however, feared that the state's use of artificial birth control as a mode of governmental regulation would fatally undermine the self-disciplining of individuals. Thus the disagreement was between those who felt that the 'common enemy', i.e. population growth, must be countered through the expansion of governmental regulation, and those who felt that the onus of this must be placed upon the individual's capacity for self-discipline. While the former argued that artificial birth control did not endanger self-discipline, and that it actually fostered it, the latter were suspicious of these claims. Viewing the debate in this way brings into focus the commonalties of these different sides, highlights the common ground of the interlocutors within the new élite, and thereby diminishes the sense of polarization.

On the national scene, however, population management: gained a new significance by the late 1950s, clearly reflected in the importance it gained within the Second Five-Year Plan (1956–60). Allocations for FP rose considerably, while health sector expenditure declined (Rao 2004: 29). This trend intensified in the Third Five-Year Plan (1961–5). Community Development initiatives were now mobilized to shift from the more passive clinic approach to the active extension approach. The FPP underwent massive expansion, with a major revamping of the machinery, in which additional posts of FP assistants, auxiliary nurse midwives, a woman doctor exclusively for FP, and the like were created (Rao 2004: 32–33). These changes were rapidly absorbed in Kerala. Within political society (in the strict Gramscian sense) too, support for FP came to be voiced more assertively. The health minister of Kerala in the late 1950s, Dr AR Menon, and other prominent members of the first communist ministry, like V.R. Krishna Aiyer, were staunch believers in the population explosion thesis and the efficacy of FP as the antidote for this malady. The period 1964–70 was one of rapid expansion of the FP machinery here, with the establishment of FP Centres statewide, and FP clinics in 93 Panchayats. Spacing methods were introduced during 1965–6 and 1967–8; incentives for promoters and doctors were boosted. Various committees were constituted at many levels for FP promotion (Beevi 1999: 231–2). Topped with full financial support from the central government, the FPP was now poised for conquest.

While these developments in the infrastructure and state support are crucial, they are not sufficient to account for the remarkable welcome granted to the entire FP project by the new Malayali élite. Nor does it reveal the ways in which the élitism of the national FPP blended smoothly into the concerns of the local élite. As detailed above, formidable suspicions were voiced quite widely in the 1930s, and these cut across sections of public opinion. Here is where some attention to other debates may prove useful. A major challenge before the advocates of artificial contraception was of finding ways to reconcile it with the sexual self-discipline of individuals: this would justify not only individual use but also the state's support for artificial birth control.

The Malayali 'Sexual Revolution'

I do not wish to argue that the remarkable change in understandings of sex and love in Malayali public discourse in the period between the 1930s and the 1960s resembled the 'sexual revolution' (Cook 2005), or even the 'permissive moment' (Weeks 1981) that historians have identified in north-west Europe and the United States around the 1960s. Indeed, it was not similar to what Weeks has discussed in the context of British society in the 1960s. The changes in the institution of marriage here seemed quite the reverse. That is, the major change seemed to be the gradual attrition of indigenous marital practices and familial arrangements that were more permissive. A hardening of conjugal marriage and the firm entrenchment of the modern gender norms structuring it, especially for large sections of people located outside the new élite, seem to have happened. Recent historical studies on the Malayali working class (Lindberg 2001) and ethnographic work on the spread of dowry practices in Malayali society (Kodoth 2006) seem to confirm this. The nuclear family form too seems to have gained considerable spread in Kerala by the mid-twentieth century (Puthenkalam 1977; Jeffrey 2003) and its ills were already being discussed in the literary public sphere by authors, for instance the rationalist–feminist K. Saraswati Amma (Devika 2002). It was against this backdrop that the cultural and social 'rehabilitation' of sex was debated and achieved.

Preceding these times was a fairly long and intense period of social and community reformist activity (Nampootiri 1999) that sought to redo family, marriage and kinship on the terms set by modern monogamous conjugality and the ideology of modern gender.[15] The need to manage the sexual activity of individuals so that it would be transformed into a resource for useful procreation had been articulated as early as the late nineteenth century. This was clearly visible in the early criticisms of the matrilineal systems of matrimonial and familial arrangements: they appeared repugnant not only because they clashed with Victorian sexual morality but also because they ostensibly failed to produce useful, healthy, and industrious progeny. Criticizing matriliny, the CMS missionary, Reverend George Mathen wrote:

> Though it is seen that the progeny of unions in which men and women live together in mutual fidelity are strong and healthy, the children of parents of easy morals are weak and sickly. And besides it is clear from the condition of the prostitutes that the immoral woman does not have the chaste wife's capacity to bear children. [Mathen [1865] 1993: 351.]

Later, the lack of proper management of sexual activity was often pointed out as underlying a perceived lack of productive habits among Malayalis. A 'Hindu Liberal' of these times wrote that 'The Malayalis are as a class the most idle and homesick of the whole Hindu community ... owing to the enervating influence exercised on their character by their peculiar system of inheritance and their obnoxious system of promiscuous marriage or no marriage at all' (*Hindu*, 6 Februay 1891, quoted in Jeffrey 1976: 6). Responses of the educated elite to the inquiries of the commission set up in Malabar in 1890 to review the condition of matrilineal marital and family practices and ascertain the possibilities of reform, confirmed these views (Arunima 2003). The respondents often referred to it as a 'prehistoric relic', rooted in a plunder-based economy, not a production-based one. This and the alleged 'sexual promiscuity' of matrilineal marriage were seen to be major obstacles to the 'progress' of the Nairs (one of the principal matrilineal communities of Kerala) (*Report of the Malabar Marriage Commission* 1891, App. iv: 1–2, 4, 7). The *Report* concluded that Malabar had not evolved out of a state of 'barbarism' because it lacked (conjugal, modern) marriage (Arunima 2003: 133). In the first Malayalam novels that appeared in these times, free-flowing sexual desire is attendant to negative qualities such as laziness, ignorance, and social and economic parasitism (Menon [1889] 1991; Nair [1890] 1988; Menon [1892] 1985).

This should be set along with the overwhelming importance granted to the 'Union of Minds' as the keystone of modern marriage within the reformist circles ever since the late nineteenth century. This was evident in the reformers' recommendation of marital and familial relationships based on 'natural feelings' and 'sentiment' to the Malabar Marriage Commission—in which the 'natural feeling' between spouses could only be romantic love (Arunima 2003: 133). The theme of the triumph of romantic love over the hurdles set by 'tradition' is central to most early nineteenth century novels in Malayalam. In these texts, *premam* (Romantic Love) is associated with animated Womanhood personified in heroines who are generally depicted as having received the correct training that has sharpened their 'inherent' capacities, and made them 'truly' womanly. In most of these, sexual intimacy is disqualified in favour of mental communion as the abiding force of stable unions. Indeed, sexual union is but a by-product of *premam*, to be reached only after the couple has experienced all the other intimacies, and is comparatively marginal as far as the stability of the union is concerned. Such unions are hailed as endowing women with active agency, enabling them to draw men into the world of emotional relationships and altruistic exchange in homely life. Romantic love was strictly delineated from *kamam*, or lust, in which women may figure only as passive victims or seductive objects. Thus, the modern conjugal unit, it was often argued, was to be held together not only by the force of the legal enactments in its favour, but by various 'internal forces', including *premam* (Devika 2007). Further, such *premam*, it was sometimes argued, could break down entrenched forms of social hierarchy. Introducing a Civil Marriages Act at the Cochin Legislative Council in 1935, the prominent reformer Sahodaran K. Ayappan spoke at length on this:

> *Premam* has a most important place in worldly life. Unnecessary barriers to *premam* must be avoided. Each person must have freedom in the matter of *premam.* To say that freedom in *premam* must be permitted does not mean that freedom in *kamam* must be allowed ... Love must be permitted to grow as freely as possible as *premam. Premam* may not respect differences of caste. [Quoted in Sanoo 1989: 151.]

Within the numerous popular novels that continued to appear right up to the 1950s, *premam* occupied centre-stage as the force emanating from fully-fledged individuals, questioning the traditional order and stabilizing the modern family (for instance, Mannadiyar 1947; Tharakan [1922] 1993; Damodaran 1947; Pillai [c.1935] 1954; Nair 1947).

Whether they permitted the 'Union of Minds' or not was a criterion used by authors to assess the implications of various reformist suggestions. Thus, in the 1930s, women reformers like Parvati Nenminimangalam expressed dissatisfaction with the suggestion that the wife should deck herself, culture her *body,* to be sexually appealing to the husband. For Nenminimangalam, it was the mind that had to be cultured; the body was to be kept minimal, shorn of its ability to arouse erotic desire in men (Nenminimangalam 1933). She was certainly not alone in her suspicion. Indeed, in most Malayali reformisms, the need to prevent exposure of the female body, so that it would not arouse carnal cravings, and thwart the project of modern self-building, was stressed (Devika 2005).

Challenges to the centrality of *premam* were however beginning to take shape even as early as the 1930s. A major, if indirect, challenge appeared from within reformist discourse centred upon the Malayala brahmin community (also referred to as the Nambutiri community reformism). Among the radical elements in Nambutiri reformism, the achievement of sexual discipline within the community clearly required a more widespread and equitable distribution of sexual activity between the sexes. V.T. Bhattatiripad, a prominent radical figure, and others, for example, were vociferous in their demands for widow-remarriage, divorce of young brahmin women married to old men, and intra-caste marriage for younger brahmin men. In defence of these demands, they inevitably pointed to the unlimited opportunities for sensual indulgence permitted to men, contrasting this to the sexual starvation of women (Bhattatiripad 1984). This was, however, firmly reined to the project of building the modern community: the sexual energy of the brahmin woman was to be tapped for the community's advance alone.[16] Further, male Malayala brahmin reformers—especially V.T. Bhattatiripad, were keen to stress that brahmin women should be reformed into efficient homemakers not only by improving their efficiency in domestic labour and management but also by accentuating their capacity to be providers of pleasure in the family. This reverberated through the discussions of dress-reform of brahmin women, in which it was argued that they needed to pick up ways of aesthetically presenting their bodies in order to keep their men (for instance, Bhattatiripad 1988: 329–39). This was also the rationale for including certain accomplishments such as singing, painting, drawing, letter writing, and etiquette in the several plans for female education that appeared in Malayali reformisms, which were to otherwise include useful skills such as cooking, home management, and childcare. In traditional Sanskritic representation of womanhood, there was a strict divide between the *kulina* and the *veshya*: she who brought forth legitimate offspring, and she who was the vessel of culture.

The ideal of the modern woman articulated in twentieth century reformisms in Malayali society is different from both these in that it combines the features of both. Woman is firmly installed within the patrilineal family and monogamous conjugality as the begetter of legitimate progeny; at the same time, she also takes over the functions of the *veshya* in a significantly different way. This is by bringing the *veshya*'s accomplishments, now thoroughly shorn of sensual flavour, into the modern home as instruments to assure the health and longevity of the modern monogamous conjugal unit. Not surprisingly, many reformers found these to be conflicting, but the debate was never resolved, and even in Malayali society of the late twentieth century, the tension remained, almost setting the terms of most discussions on women's space and freedom (Devika 2005; 2006). Even as mind-centred *premam* was being hailed as the central pivot of the modern conjugal unit, the simultaneous assignment of the role of 'provider of pleasure' to the wife—this 'fault-line' at the core of the ideal of modern womanhood in Kerala—left open a loop-hole. Through this it became possible to assert that the sustenance of pleasure-generation within the family was absolutely necessary if its stability was to be ensured. This was subsequently advanced as a key argument to establish the necessity of artificial birth control as an important instrument in preserving the pleasurableness of the monogamous conjugal union. It also helped defeat the plea that the shift towards pleasure that artificial birth control might allow would potentially damage disciplined family life, pointing to the possibility that if the wife eschewed her role as the provider of pleasure to the husband, he might seek it elsewhere.

Secondly, the solidity of *premam* was being questioned in the fast-expanding domain of modern Malayalam literature, in the 'literary public sphere'—one in which social issues were closely debated, albeit mediated by fictional narratives, for instance, Changampuzha Krishna Pillai's *Ramanan* (1936). Here we need to note that the breadth and reach of the literary public in Kerala was growing at a tremendous pace in these very decades. It was fuelled by the remarkable expansion of popular literacy in these decades: literacy rates in Travancore and Cochin rose from 24.2

and 18.5 per cent in 1921 to 47.1 and 41.0 in 1941 (Jeffrey 2003: 57). In Malabar, literacy rates jumped from 14.4 in 1931 to 30.9 per cent in 1951. The expansion of the literary reading public is also evident in the large number of journals in which these debates were featured. Often, these debates occurred as part of larger discussions around the relevance of particular political ideologies, especially Marxism, and were then reprinted as pamphlets and discussed by party-members—for instance, V.T. Induchoodan's *Kalayum Marxisavum* (Art and Marxism) and M.S. Devadas's *Premavum Purogamanasahityavum* (Love and Progressive Literature) (Chandrasekharan 1999: 30). Many of the authors discussed were astoundingly popular for instance Changampuzha Krishna Pillai, whose pastoral elegy, *Ramanan,* was widely discussed. In 1945, the noted critic Joseph Mundassery wrote thus, hinting that this text introduced a cross-section of people to reading: 'For some time now, *Ramanan* has been Lesson One in the beach and balcony, the boat-jetty and the bus station, the temple-kitchens and bungalows, huts, fields, factories and army barracks' (Mundassery 1955: 25). Besides, in the 1930s, both the community movements, and the nationalist and communist movements used literature as a powerful medium for propaganda, and several reformers and politicians often doubled up as song writers, story-writers, playwrights, or actors for their movements (Jeffery 2003: 134–35). For instance, the Malayala brahmin reformers V.T. Bhattatiripad and M.R. Bhattiripad, and communist leaders like Thoppil Bhasi and K. Damodaran wrote short stories and plays. Poets like Vallathol Narayana Menon espoused the nationalist cause. Thus the debates within this arena had considerable impact, with continually widening circles of readership.

Modernists in Malayalam were major initiators of the debate on *premam* and *kamam*, and the noted modernist intellectual Kesari A. Balakrishna Pillai took a lead here. Indeed, he was often the target of conservative criticism, which accused him of having let loose 'futuristic' ideas that allegedly transformed his younger followers into advocates of sexual anarchy (Sastry 1948). In his 'Biographical Notes', written towards the end of the 1940s, he observed, in retrospect, 'I do not regard the sex life of man as the mean portion of his nature. A sex-impulse is as natural and noble as another so-called noble impulse. This is why I showed tolerance for sexual feeling in man' (appended to Sukumaran 1987: 199–213). Intellectuals began to express scepticism about the now familiar ways of regulating sexual desire, ranging from the use of discreet language and modest dress, to mind-centred *premam* as a regulatory force toning down *kamam,* and making it subservient to modern domesticity. All covering and dressing of the female body, it was pointed out, was a double-edged sword; it aroused as much desire as it prevented (Thomas 1953: 19–25). Another author remarked that *premam*, under highly constraining social conditions, could only be a flimsy excuse for lust. Hence, only if women and men were allowed to enjoy 'sexual freedom in life' would the 'real' *premam* (which was attributed the capacity to bind together men and women) flourish (Karippaayi 1939: 23). The Progressive Writers were sceptical about *premam*, which they sought either to discredit or redefine in unique ways. Thus we find sexual desire partially rehabilitated as *Hridayattinte Vishappu* (The Hunger of the Heart) in Ponkunnam Varkey's short story challenging the exclusive identification of *premam* and the 'heart': its title became the target of much criticism as expressing the rehabilitation of desire. Indeed, one of the major criticisms earned by the so-called 'Progressive Writers' of mid-twentieth century in Kerala was that they were producing lewd writing in the name of realistic portrayal (Sastry 1948: 154; for an overview of the debates, Chandrasekharan 1999). In the writings of those commonly viewed as 'Progressive Writers' in Malayalam (Takazhi Sivasankara Pillai, P. Kesavadev, Ponkunnam Varkey, Vaikam Muhammad Basheer, and others) one finds on the one hand texts critical of the hypocrisy that renders sexual desire invisible and mute, and on the other, texts that sharply criticize the 'sexual excesses' of the rich that make impossible the fostering of sentimental affection and bourgeois familial values among the poor. In short, it seems difficult to characterize the Progressive writers as unambiguous opponents of 'bourgeois' sexual morality. At the same time, it may be admitted that their writing, in these times, was taken to represent the 'freeing' of sexuality from bourgeois prudery and hypocrisy.[17]

However, even when the short stories of writers like Takazhi Sivasankara Pillai, Kesavadev, and Ponkunnam Varkey departed sharply from the literary conventions attending body-less *premam*, their spokespersons rebutted charges of 'sexual indiscipline' levelled against them in debates. M.P. Paul, in his speech at the Progressive Writers' conference at Thrissur, declared that while the Progressive Writers could not shut their eyes to sexuality, they would have to guard against excesses (Chandrasekharan 1999). The well-known poet and intellectual of the forties, Changampuzha Krishna Pillai, in his celebrated address to a meeting of the Progressive Writers in 1945, criticized prudery about sex in literature, and critics who refused to see excess of sexual description in Sanskrit texts and traditional literary genres. He, however, called for more efficient ways of regulating desire:

> Those who are interested in the morality of the future generation should not seek to childishly conceal such terms as the above [the reference was to the word 'mula' which means 'breast' in Malayalam] in asterisks; rather the effort should be to impart sex-education from an early age.' [Pillai 1953: 71–2.]

Leftist writers either tried to articulate a 'proletarian critique' of *premam*, often condemning the Progressive Writers' challenge as 'decadent'. Their criticisms of the latter certainly reeked of Victorian sexual values (for instance, Devadas [1949] 1991; Nambutiripad [1949] 1999: 282–96; [1949a] 1999: 336–45), but they remained suspicious of the capacity of 'bourgeois' *premam* as a force capable of channelling the sexual energies of individuals in a productive way. Instead they sought to install Reason as the appropriate 'internal force' sealing modern conjugality (for instance, Devadas [1949] 1991; Pisharady 1971, 1981) and projecting marriage as a relationship 'for mating and making a living through labour' (Devadas [1949] 1991: 33). In other words, their thrust was not so much on rejecting *premam* wholesale, as on redoing it and installing Reason at its heart, and opening up a certain, if more closely-watched, space for lust. Sexual desire was acknowledged, in a scaled-down version, as a 'physical need' that had necessarily to be met if people were to lead 'normal' lives. A sharp distinction was drawn between 'animal' and 'human' forms of desire; comparisons were drawn between humankind's constant efforts not just to control Nature but to harness it to human needs; a universal theory of human history was evoked to prove the point. Drawing on Christopher Caudwell, the prominent communist critic, M.S. Devadas argued thus:

> [Caudwell establishes that] Since we do not let our emotions run loose or allow them to scatter, like the savages of the old—since we keep our 'natural emotions' more under control, under 'repression'—we are able to satiate our emotions and our desires better ... That is, the very emotional life of modern man is many times superior to that of the primitive man in the cultural values that it is endowed with. Our love is not merely lust; it is a new type of female–male relationship that is more stable, focused and firm. [Devadas [1949] 1991: 61.]

Hence the importance granted to monogamous marriage as an institution that helped to meet this need in a socially non-disruptive manner. This fresh stress on Reason and self-discipline also flowed from other sources, for example, the rationalist movement that was becoming a conspicuous presence since the 1930s, represented in the public by such eminent reformers as Sahodaran K. Ayappan and 'Yuktivadi' K.C. Joseph. K.C. Joseph, for instance, was keen on pointing to the need to refurbish marriage on a 'scientific basis': which began with scepticism towards the efficacy of *premam* as an instrument assuring the longevity of the institution. Instead, he recommended rational consideration of all factors, and especially self-discipline (Sanoo 2002: 119). *Yuktivadi*, the well-known rationalist journal that he edited, stressed the need for rational control of the intellect over the emotions (Sanoo 2002: 208). Another prominent rationalist and popular author, Kuttipuzha Krishna Pillai too pointed out that marriages were sustained not by *premam* but by financial stability (Pillai [1965] 1990: 152–5). These intellectuals were largely liberals, often left-leaning, and as in the West, their endorsement of birth control was born from their faith that humanity was on the brink of a major leap ahead in the control of suffering through science and technological change, and that the major impediment to this was organized religion (Dowbiggin 2002).

Premam also faced similar attack from other quarters, such as the rationalist–feminism of K. Saraswati Amma. She too sought to redraw *premam* as the union of rational minds capable of discarding gender difference. She, however, considered such unions to be the rarest in contemporary times, which were not conducive to the self-development of individuals, especially women, into fully individuated persons. Also, Saraswati Amma shrewdly pointed out that in order to fully realize Reason-centred *premam* as a force assuring the stability of the marital bond, women must be allowed to 'flirt'; to freely mingle with men, so that they may be able to rationally decide upon suitable mates! (Amma 1955). *Premam,* in the form that was popular in those times, was faulted for its sentimentality, and for the fact that it seemed to have lost the subversive energies once attributed to it (as, for example, in the challenge it raised to the established orders by enabling inter-caste marriages) (Devika 2003).

Not surprisingly, sex-education figured as the major instrument for inculcating sexual self-discipline, and this seemed more or less agreed upon by all these different participants in the debates. Changampuzha's famous defence of the Progressive Writers (quoted above) mentioned it. Saraswati Amma recommended it, finding that it relied upon modern science to generate truth about the human body, apparently crucial for disciplining one's bodily desires. Devadas waxed eloquent about sex-education in the USSR. Arguing that Soviet society promoted 'intellectual' and 'legitimate' friendships between men and women, he noted:

> Since [asexual, 'legitimate'] friendships are allowed to grow between boys and girls from childhood, and because they receive knowledge about the seriousness of sexual life early, there is no encouragement of sexual perversions like masturbation among the Soviet youth. As masturbation is considered harmful from the point of view of health for the masculinity of boys and the femininity of girls and psychologically, it is capable of breeding excessive egoism, it is considered a despicable perversion that should be prohibited. [Devadas [1949] 1991: 66–7.]

The call for sex-education in Kerala appears to date back to the 1920s. The earliest texts that I could find were published from Kottayam and written by V.C. John (1929; 1930). A landmark work detailing contemporary scientific thinking on human sexuality, Nalappatt Narayana Menon's *Ratisamrajyam,* was published in 1938, and widely circulated. In the 1940s, several texts purporting to provide scientific information on sex and desire were published, some widely read, like Helen Thomas' *Dambatyapremam* (Love in Marriage) (1945) and *Jananiyantranam* (Birth Control) (1948). Sex-education was being recommended as a prerequisite for introducing artificial birth control by legislators like V. Gangadharan Nair in 1951 (*Proceedings of the Travancore–Cochin Legislative Assembly* 1952: 1594). Numerous articles stressing the need for sex-education in the 1930s and '40s, and a flood of texts came in the 1950s and '60s.[18] P.M. Mathew's *Kumarikumaranmarute Prasnangal* (The problems of adolescent boys and girls), serialized in the *Malayala Manorama* (*MM*) in 1967, was widely welcomed. However, criticisms were still to be heard in the 1950s, and not necessarily from Catholics (for instance, Menon [1955] 1970). 'Sex-education' ended up as a convenient label for soft-porn films made in Malayalam but it is significant that this label is used for their justification. This involved more than knowledge of human physiology. Indeed, the human mind too was being viewed often as full of 'secrets' that might only be unravelled by scientific inquiry. Writing on the 'secret corridors' of the minds, accessible only through the penetrating gaze of modern science began to appear from the 1940s onwards.[19]

A point on which the different champions of sex-education could agree was regarding the source and direction of the flow of information about sexual matters: that it should originate from science and flow from the expert to the layperson. Such demands were made early enough of marriage-and-family guides to distinguish them from texts that offered guidance in the erotic arts, which were inevitably dismissed as prurient and polluting (for instance, Kurup 1928: iii). The former did not entirely distance themselves from earlier models of *Kamasastra* texts or from traditional prescriptions for obtaining healthy offspring (for instance, Menon 1929; 1930; Nambutiri 1929). The demand for a scientific attitude in speaking about sexual affairs became more insistent subsequently on, and authors were careful to mention their commitment to the scientific and objective viewpoint in their books; reviewers congratulated authors for adhering to the scientific spirit in their writing (Narayanan [1952] 1960: 219; *Kerala Kaumudi* (henceforth, *KK*) 4 April 1971: 5; *MM* 24 September 1967: 4). Ideally, all speech and writing regarding sexual matters were to be couched in objective and scientific language, and to flow from the expert to the layperson, so that no lascivious feelings were aroused that could block the scientific self-gaze of the latter. Also, the ability to view the issues scientifically, it was argued, permitted 'openness'; this was sometimes interpreted as heightening pleasure (Udayabhanu 1965). This was certainly not new; the same expectation regarding sex education existed elsewhere: for instance, in the sex-education initiatives undertaken by women reformers in the US in the 1920s and 1930s. Similar hopes that sex-education would rescue people from 'excessive indulgence' and 'carnality', coupled with strong objections to commercial sex and pornography, existed in these efforts. However, the difference is also significant: while in the US, these gave the opportunity for some public discussion on female sexuality and pleasure, even though controversially and with much opposition from within the ranks (Wheeler 2000), here, women participants in the debates were few. The two authors who did participate—Saraswati Amma and Lalitambika Antarjanam—were either ignored or promptly silenced (Devika 2003; Raveendran n.d: 82). A later and more powerful intervention, Madhavikutty's autobiographical *Ente Katha* (My Story) was completely absorbed into late modernism in Malayalam, with its subversion completely effaced (Devika 2006a). In general, sex-education texts depicted women principally as the possessors of a largely procreative sexuality, though Nalappatt Narayana Menon did bring in a more extended discussion in *Ratisamrajyam*.

The above mentioned features found desirable for proper sex-education were especially pronounced in the texts that began to be produced and actively circulated by the Catholic Church. The vast literature on sexual life and self-discipline produced by the Catholic Church in the 1960s attempted a combination of sex-education with *premam* (here it figured merely as an internal force cementing the conjugal unit, and not as one capable of breaking down distinctions of class or caste) in which both are deemed equally important in assuring the productive regulation of sexual desire (for instance, see Ponnookkara 1979; 1979a; Jose 1975; 1970; 1971; Kalappura 1972; Manikkathan 1972; 1973). These books too had considerable circulation: *Avan Valarunnu* (He is Growing), first published in 1966, went into its sixth edition in 1979, as did *Aval Valarunnu* (She is Growing) and *Dambatyajeevitattiloode* (Through Conjugal Life). However, even in this literature it seemed no more possible to treat sexual desire as easily subjugated to sentimental attachments. *Premam* no longer seemed prior to *kamam* in importance; once its ineffectuality in regulating the latter seemed evident, other means were to be sought. More and more frequently, the sexual urge is admitted to be a fundamental structuring element of the human mind, and not easily socialized. Thus, in the writings of Catholic sex educators, while sex was accepted to be part of the positive side of God's creation, it was to be strictly shaped according to 'God's plan'. Drawing upon the then pervasive language of centralized planning and development, Dr Louis Ponnookkara, author of *Avan Valarunnu*, wrote:

> God has deposited in men and women unique tendencies and emotions that draw them into conjugal life. But all those are permitted only within the plan God has decided upon. Only then will the blessing 'multiply and thrive' [and] become complete. But there are tendencies to act outside [the plan] ... Sex is a beautiful reality within God's plan. If sex is taken outside God's plan, it becomes ugly. As a necessary effect of this, society, too, becomes ugly.... [Ponnookkara 1979: 13–5.]

The further recommendations specify who the agents of sex-education are to be and what the content must be. Besides, most clearly, sex-education was to affirm gender difference as an important tool to make young boys and girls comfortable with the ideal subjectivities that appeared 'naturally' implied in their respective sexual endowments. The author lays special emphasis on the necessity of priests taking up the responsibility of imparting such education about 'God's plan', 'given the contemporary atmosphere', and criticizes nuns who who have 'not yet escaped the clutches of the Manichean devil, that sex is evil' (Ponnookkara 1979: 17). He however remembers that the enlightened among the nuns have indeed 'indirectly taken up the exalted task of preparing every young girl for marriage, with maternal affection' (Ponnookkara 1979: 17–18). The content he insists, should not be merely physiology, but a mixture of psychology and physiology, but in his account there is a load of moral advice, which is heavier than either of these. Indeed, he refrains from any explicit description of the sexual act, and indeed, warns against others who may provide it to the child: namely, 'servants, friends and prurient writings' (Ponnookkara 1979: 23; 84–5).

Thus, notwithstanding their many (and noisily expressed) differences, publicists of different persuasions often converged upon sex-education as a major means of regulating carnal desires. As indicated above, there were several variants, more conservative or less. However, the agreement upon the necessity to channel sexual energies productively ensured the retention of a sexual morality classifying sexual behaviour into 'good' and 'bad' types. Bodily desires now gained admittance as a 'basic need', that simultaneously allowed an equally strict, if less conspicuous form of regulation. Secondly, sex-education was also a powerful tool of modern gendering: it was most often viewed as an instrument affirming gender difference, and drew actively upon the by-then highly familiar ideology of modern gender.

What is significant to us here is this: the consecration of sexual desire at the heart of modern conjugal union alongside or even above *premam*, it may be argued, helped to open up further the 'fault-line' that already ran through the modern ideal of womanhood as it was shaped in early Malayali modernity. This, I believe, was of crucial importance in making possible the effective presentation of the case for family planning in Malayali society by the 1960s, for it implied that artificial birth control was indeed a necessity for chaste wives who wished to stabilize their marriages.

Making sexual pleasure an important condition for assuring the stability of the modern conjugal unit implied that more reliable methods of contraception were inevitable. Under economic circumstances that made the sustenance of a large family difficult (widely perceived to be existing in Malayali society in those times), the non-availability of reliable birth control methods, it was argued, would make it impossible for women to be pleasure-giving mates, and that men would seek illicit sex to satisfy their desires not being bound by anatomy, as women were. Self-control, it now seemed, had to be reframed. Remarking on the relationship between artificial birth control and sexual self-control, an author wrote:

> It may be remembered that self-control and birth control are not solutions that may be substituted for one another. Self-control may be essential irrespective of whether one uses artificial birth control methods or not. It is dangerous to practice asceticism through abstention from sex for very long. The moral danger is that there will be the temptation to indulge in sex with someone outside. For oneself, even the mutual relation may be endangered. [Kurien 1958: 71.]

The same text admitted that unmarried persons might 'misuse' artificial birth control to indulge in the pleasures of the flesh, but this was met with the argument that self-control was necessary, irrespective of whether or not one used artificial birth control techniques. The very same fears were voiced after the Papal rejection of artificial birth control in 1968. In 1969, the Catholic Church held the Kerala Regional Seminar at Aluva in which the problems of conjugality and faith were actively raised, and the Church's stand regarding artificial birth control came under sharp criticism. Several speakers affirmed the centrality of conjugal *premam* to be equally important as sex-education in regulating sexual desire, but opinions were certainly not unanimous, and differences in positions were vociferously argued. Indeed, the argument regarding the centrality of sex in conjugal stability was evoked precisely in defence of artificial contraception (Joseph 1972: 136–53). P.C. Chacko, a speaker at the public meeting that followed the seminar, made this link clear, forcefully arguing that sex was indeed fundamental to the stability of marital union, and to treat it as marginal would be to encourage 'wanderings': 'In marriage, procreation is not the sole aim of sexual union. Union in marriage is a lifetime association. Sexual union is a fundamental element in a stable marital union ... sex is the link that binds the mother and the father.' (quoted in Joseph 1972: 153). He further pointed out that the demand for artificial contraception may be regarded as the product of love and concern shared by the conjugal couple—the husband's concern for the health of the wife, their mutual concern for the children—and not merely as an outcome of their carnal cravings (Joseph 1972: 155).

Though Catholic magazines like *Amma* obsessively pursued the themes of the stability of the modern conjugal marriage and the nuclear household, they were indeed general concerns in these times. By the mid-1950s and 1960s, it began to be observed that the emergent institution of modern marriage resembled not the sublime union of minds, but a crass and materialistic financial transaction. Nowhere is this documented so well as in K. Saraswati Amma's short stories, which sketch the emergent institution with brilliant unsentimental insight (Ravikumar 2000). Academic observers have also closely recorded the spread of the system of dowry payments into more and more communities in Malayali society precisely around this period (Puthenkulam 1977; Lindberg 2001; Osella and Osella 2001). Besides, the difficult problem of integrating two different fully-fledged *individuals* in gender-mediated altruistic exchange within the familial institution to constitute a smoothly functioning unit loomed large. Magazines exclusively devoted to the health of the family were not new—for instance, *Sumangala* (1916) was devoted to equipping householders and homemakers for their respective tasks, but the shift towards more psychological themes on the same topic and later family magazines such as, for instance *Kudumbapatrik*a of the 1930s, is striking. Later, the 'adjustment problems' of working mothers' carrying the double burden began to be discussed.[20] Indeed, the search for ways of ensuring the longevity of modern marriage would have appeared all the more urgent in the face of these emergent tensions.

Thus, by the 1960s, a strong case was made for the rehabilitation of sex within the conjugal union, which also made a case for artificial contraception within it. It became possible to argue that artificial contraception was not contrary to the project of self-disciplining; in fact, the possibility of arguing that artificial birth control aided the self-disciplining of individuals was now open. The concern about finding ways of ensuring the stability of modern marriage and family was also becoming fairly pervasive. The intensive FP campaign of the 1960s thrived upon these shifts; they virtually provided the very foundations of its ideological structure. It built upon these, assiduously sharing the concerns expressed about the social regulation of sexual activity in the interests of the modern family and the development-fixated modern nation. Thus, its agents were only-too anxious to project themselves as fully committed to the maintenance of 'family values' and 'dharma', and to point out that the safer methods were strictly limited to married persons (for instance, editorial, *Matrubhumi* 18 December 1966: 4). FP propagandists were never tired of exhorting the public not to put artificial contraception to 'immoral' use. The speech delivered by the Kerala state health minister, B. Wellington, at the inauguration of the condom factory at Thiruvananthapuram, is just one such instance. As *Kerala Kaumudi* reported it:

> The Health Minister B. Wellington stated that a transformation in sexual life that parallels those in the socio–economic and political fields is necessary. He reminded that the instruments of Family Planning were not to be used to create unregulated sexual anarchy. He stated that the movement, which was the product of the good intention of establishing the stability of society, should not become a license for moral deterioration. [*KK* 6 April, 1969: 7.]

As for abortions, the FP propagandists reminded their critics that the call to legalize abortions fully recognized the need for the social regulation of sexual activity in the interests of the family, and that it certainly did not grant women any real control over their reproductive capacities. Dr C.O. Karunakaran, one of the foremost FP propagandists in Kerala defended legalizing abortions thus:

> No one has demanded unregulated abortions. The suggestion is that if a woman with more than two or three children demands abortion with the consent of her husband and out of economic reasons, there should be no legal barrier. Besides, she will have to consent to sterilization in order to prevent any later pregnancies. [*KK* 11 August 1967: 2.]

The pro-familial image of the FPP was nurtured in more ways than one. A 'positive image' was sought to be created, and the propaganda often claimed that FP services were not reducible to sterilization but also included treatment of sterility (for instance, Velayudhan 1967; Nair 1971; Oommen 1966; Peetambaran 1969: 88). That artificial birth control was intended only for married couples was never sufficiently underscored: at an FP propaganda seminar at the Recreation Club of the Alind Industries, Kundara, entry was prohibited to unmarried persons below eighteen years of age (*MM* 11 September 1959: 4). This went along with the claim that using FP methods would greatly increase conjugal happiness by permitting carefree intercourse, thereby ensuring its permanence. 'Openness' and 'freedom' were sought, but within the limits of the monogamous family, and strictly bound to productivist imperatives. As A.P. Udayabhanu, another visible FP enthusiast, exclaimed 'I can guarantee that after this (i.e. undergoing vasectomy), life has been 'free of fear', 'contented' and 'anxiety-less'. After the operation, husband and wife stopped fearing each other'. As for the effect, '... "Enthusiasm" may be heightened a bit. It is said that old men practice this to gain youth' (Udayabhanu 1970).

Moreover, the FPP shared the language of sex-education in which sexual matters could be spoken of 'objectively', and thus clearly distanced itself from the charge of being prurient. Even the Catholic critics of the intensive FPP of the early 1970s found fault with it not on the ground that it would heighten the appetite for sex, but in that it seemed to be altogether against children (Joseph 1972: 31–2). In general, early FP propaganda tended to emphasize economic hardships and social failings of large families in explicit terms, and couched its implications for the sexual life of couples in much more veiled language. This was, in fact, praised by commentators as one of the reasons for the success of FP propaganda in the 1960s. Reviewing the much-staged FP propaganda play *Sandhi,* M.P. Manmathan remarked:

> Propagating awareness of the problem on a large scale but limiting the knowledge of its solution to those of the right age and in a private manner—that is the practical and intelligent way to popularize family planning. To deviate from this balance, and make propaganda the naked and public popularization of birth control methods, will not only prevent the realization of desired results but also lead us to sexual anarchy. [*Matrubhumi* 14 April 1967: 1.]

Sandhi was praised for giving just a hint of the contraceptives while highlighting the woes of large families. Soon however the FP propagandists were quite willing to go further and publicize the various methods of artificial contraception. Once dealt with 'scientifically', all sexual matters could be easily spoken of in public, the adoption of a 'scientific' posture being a necessary condition for the propagation of artificial birth control. This was part of the FPP from early days, and continued to be demanded (Narayanan 1960: 218–19; Peetambaran 1968: 89). The prestige of the scientific language gave FP propagandists the confidence to unleash an all-out campaign to break through the barriers of social reticence. When shrewdly implemented, this could yield rich rewards for the population controllers, as the chief organizer of the much-publicized mass sterilization camps at Ernakulam in the early 1970s, S. Krishna Kumar testified:

> The camp succeeded also in large measure in overcoming the resistance to the adoption of vasectomy as a family planning method resulting from a feeling of embarrassment of the male born out of the fear of others knowing of the operation and in general from the prudery regarding a subject relating to sex and reproduction. The Town Hall at the very centre of the town was selected as the venue for the camp and the camp was organized in full public gaze with the aim of breaking through this barrier. Though for the first few days this resistance could be felt it was progressively overcome....

> The prospective acceptors could be seen standing in queue in front of the operation room as casually and without any self-consciousness as if they were at a cinema ticket-counter [Kumar 1971: 65–7.]

The public slogans stressed the importance of family limitation to the progress of the nation, and FP as the duty of the patriotic citizen. The slogans raised in the FP rally organized in connection with the camp were: 'Hear the voices of the Indian masses/Who sweat and toil on this sacred land/Hear this patriotic clarion call/ Two [parents] we are, and two [children] for us' (Kumar 1971: 67). Meanwhile, 'private' and 'personal' objections were dealt with in sheltered domains. About the door-to-door campaign of the camp of 1971, he says: 'Each prospective promotee had personal and complicated reasons for his attitude to family planning and this type of field organisation and work ensured the personalised attention that was necessary to take him to a decision-making stage.' Such work, he said, '... delves deeply into the psychological barriers' that stood in the way of FP adoption (Kumar 1971: 106).

However, the 'openness' that seems to have been created seemed, at best, ambiguous. Jubilant claims were made by the Malayalam press during the mass sterilization camps of the 1970s that sterilization was now out in the open; no longer a closeted affair. The editorial of the *Matrubhumi* exulted: 'Until recently, vasectomy was prevalent among us only as a protective and private measure adopted here and there by some folks. [but in the Ernakulam camp] ... The reticence of individuals and society towards vasectomy has ended' (22 December 1970). Knowledge-Action-Practice studies from the 1950s to the early '70s have shown a spread of the circle of conversation as far as contraceptive practices are concerned (GoK 1978: 88–90). Nonetheless the divide between the 'scientific' language of managing sex, and the 'ordinary' language of expressing 'forbidden pleasures', which offers a choice between equally objectifying alternatives, is very much alive. Too much cannot be read into the exultation about the arrival of' 'openness' either. A survey conducted in ten villages in Kerala in 1983–4 revealed overwhelming support for FP, to the rather disturbing extent that '... people are really frightened of the prospect of a large family' (Varghese 1986: 166–70). This, however, does not seem to have driven the people into 'openness': 'However villagers do not like it to be known that they use contraceptives and so they buy it in other villages or towns where they are not known ...' (Varghese 1986: 167–8). In any case, there is some evidence to suggest that often, when 'openness' seems to have incarnated, it came in the form of a subtle coercion, a norm forcing people to submit even when they do not feel the need for it. The anthropologist Marion den Uyl, working in the Sachivottamapuram Colony in the 1980s, notes that the decision to accept FP by any member of that community is almost invariably preceded by an open discussion; she also notes that it has become 'a generally accepted norm' (den Uyl 1995: 181–3), so strong that there is social pressure on those who did not immediately endorse it. More recent investigations only reveal the huge ignorance about contraception in general and the available options, especially among women. The use of temporary methods, like elsewhere in India, is not popular, and researchers have noted considerable ignorance regarding those (Zachariah et al. 1994: 129). There is also indication that abortions have increased in Kerala, which may tell us that unwanted pregnancies are quite frequent (Rajan et al. 2000). Indeed, even now, safe sex, contraceptive choices or sexual/reproductive health remain matters that are not fully public. Very recently, the shadow of AIDS has led to the promotion of sex education in schools. However, the taboos it appears are still strong. In their report on gender in democratic decentralization in contemporary Kerala, Aleyamma Vijayan and J. Sandhya mention an incident in which the chairperson of the women's welfare committee, which had advanced a proposal for a unit to produce cheap and affordable sanitary napkins, had to walk out of the panchayat committee meeting in protest, as she was accused of having suggested a 'vulgar' and 'obscene' proposal. (Vijayan and Sandhya 2004: 47).

The New Missionaries

I have argued that shaping a certain qualified openness regarding sexual matters (in scientific language, in the interests of a productive society and nation, enabling governmental intervention and social regulation of individual sexuality through the monogamous, patrifocal modern family) contributed to the success of the FPP in Malayali society. However, population management certainly involved more than this, touching upon important social axes of power such as class and gender. The FPP rhetoric certainly did not attempt any radical upset of existent power equations. Indeed, the division between the 'educated' and the 'respectable', the worthy subjects of development, voluntarily committing themselves to it, and the 'masses', the stragglers (who for that reason sometimes seemed to need some shoving around), was reinforced. At the same time, the FPP appeared to be the apolitical solution to political questions, primarily inhabiting the domain of the 'social'. Indeed, the solutions that it proposed may broadly be termed 'familial', in that it appeared as though questions of unequal access to power and resources may be resolved from within the family, or at least that a beginning was to be made from within the family.

Neo-Malthusianism has been widely criticized for unjustifiably whipping up a veritable hysteria over the increase in human numbers in the survival of life on earth, effectively obscuring the highly uneven consumption and distribution of resources and global geopolitics (Mamdani 1976: 1141–48; Nadkarni 1976: 1163–73; Banerjee 1985; Rao 2004). The sceptics of various political persuasions: Catholics (for instance, *ND* 15 January 1932: 6; *ND* 21 June 1936; *ND* 13 November 1951; editorial, *ND* 24 May 1956; *ND* 17 May 1959; *ND* 22 May 1960), communists, and others voiced this critique in public in the mid-twentieth century. In the debate over FP in the Travancore–Cochin legislature of 1951, the communist member E. Gopalakrishna Menon strongly expressed such objections (*Proceedings of the Travancore–Cochin Legislative Assembly* 1952: 1601–3). Later, in 1957, E.M.S. Nambutiripad intervened in a hostile exchange in the Kerala Legislative Assembly between P.T. Chacko and V.R. Krishna Aiyer (sceptic and defender of FP respectively), to clarify that the Communist Party 'welcomed Family Planning for health reasons. The Party does not consider Family Planning to be a solution to the problems that confront us today' (*ND* 20 June 1957: 1). While agreeing with some of the rationales made for FP by the population control establishment, leftists were loath to concede too much to the effectiveness of FP as an instrument of development (Sukumaran 1963; Nambutiripad 1963; Nambutiripad, speech, reported in *KK* 17 April 1967: 2). In a speech in support of the FPP in 1967, E.M.S. Nambutiripad went so far as to agree with the then-fashionable claim that a reduction in numbers would lower the social welfare burdens of the state and help capital accumulation, but the centrality of population as the factor inducing underdevelopment was never conceded (*Matrubhumi* 27 September 1967: 3).[21] Thus, when FP propagandists complained that the support offered by the communists was not wholehearted (Chandrasekhar 1966: 68–71; Karunakaran 1967; editorial, *KK* 11 March 1967), it was the concern over the uneven distribution of wealth and resources that was being criticized as idle nit-picking.

The FP propaganda, however, remained largely insulated from such reservations and qualifications made by the communists. An apolitical explanation of poverty and want, and an apolitical solution to these dovetailed neatly within the FP propaganda. C.O. Karunakaran's downright apolitical understanding of the poverty and misery of Tamil people being shipped off to Malaya as plantation labour is a particularly interesting instance. The sight of the wretched poor he had seen being bundled off as 'labour' to be underpaid, abused, and grossly insulted is mentioned to have awakened in him a zeal for birth control (Karunakaran 1967). It does not however even seem necessary to inquire after the historical and political conditions that shaped such a state of affairs. Indeed, no explanation is offered at all; only a solution in which an explanation is already implied: 'people who cannot be fed and given work should not be born at all' (Karunakaran 1967). Interestingly, he also recommended a series of penal measures, such as denying medical and other benefits to families that did not conform to the ideal size determined by the statisticians and the bureaucrats. The burden of the solution is neatly placed upon the shoulders of the self-disciplined, industrious, enlightened *individual*. When the root cause of the problem was said to be located within oneself, and well within one's volition, then the solution may also be easily taken to be one of acting upon oneself. In case of resistance (which would, in this scheme of things, be irrational), a benevolent state committed to general welfare would be justified in introducing measures that would leave compliance the only option. A more nuanced understanding of colonialism and its compulsions, changes in the agrarian structure, transformation in rural social life, and the like in the question of 'excess labour' would have hardly legitimized the identification of the breeding habits of the poor as primarily responsible for their condition.

Thus, a major issue in poverty alleviation, it seemed, was how to make 'ignorant' individuals see the 'truth': that their situation was primarily a product of their lack of enlightenment and lack of initiative. Highlighting the tremendous social danger and individual disadvantage stemming from such irresponsibility was one key propaganda strategy. This was built on constructing a series of contrasting models of 'progress' and 'doom'; 'enlightened' supporters and 'superstitious' objectors; the few fit for self-control and the 'masses' unfit for it. Incidentally, everyone feared the 'masses': objectors, who felt that artificial birth control may be 'misused' by them, and supporters who feared the consequence of not making them accept artificial birth control one way or the other. This was of course central to eugenics-oriented pleas for sterilization, not infrequent in the early debates over artificial birth control, such as those made by Travancore legislators like P. Kunjukrishnan and Kadakkavur P. Madhavan in 1938 and 1945 respectively (*Proceedings of the Travancore Sree Mulam* 1939: 803; *Proceedings of the Travancore Sree Mulam Assembly* 1946a: 281). However, more ingenious ways of firming the divide were invented by the 1960s, through which FP was 'normed' into the individual psyche. For instance, there was the divide posited between Malayalis who lived up to their image of being 'progressive', and those who did not. The *Kerala Kaumudi* was particularly insistent on this: it repeatedly urged all Malayalis to live up to their progressive image by accepting FP (see editorials, *KK* 21 June 1967; 24 September 1967; 28 July 1968; 19 December 1968; 13 December 1969; 12 July 1970; 28 October 1971). The inferiority of those who inhabited the space below the line was reiterated in many ways, and in a number of different quarters. Large families were deemed to be filthy: writing about the necessity of birth control, a propagandist wrote: 'How many houses and courtyards with very many dirty and screaming children infested with scabies and eczema, almost indistinguishable by age, adorn our rural scene!' (Narayanan 1960: 29). Commending the work of FP, the well-known author Lalitambika Antarjanam wrote that women should emulate the elephant that gives birth only once in twelve years, and not the pig that delivers a number of young every year, to be thrown 'into the dirty gutters' (*KK* 22 July 1971: 5). Large families were apparently unhappy, unloved, and discontented (*KK* 19 December 1968: 6; *KK* 18 October 1970: 8; *KK Sunday Magazine* 5 April 1970: 6). They were also condemned as a threat to public decency and individual privacy. This was particularly a topic harnessed to evoke derisive laughter; authors of humorous articles wrote on how large families disturbed others, raided others' pockets (Krishnankutty 1961: 52–6). They were also apparently hellholes of female slavery (Karunakaran 1967a). They were the very seats of privation and ignorance, above all, an unbearable burden for both their members as well as the state responsible for their well-being. The Progressive writer P. Kesavadev wrote a whole novel, *Njana Tettukaran* (I am the One at Fault), which drew lurid pictures of such families (Vasantan 1986: 79–80). During the mass sterilization camp at Ernakulam in July 1971, a tableau was prominently taken out on a jeep depicting a large family full of miserable and emaciated-looking children, with a banner screaming, 'Let This Misery Not Happen To You' (Kumar 1971: 105). The theme of a starved ever-growing population being a political threat was evoked by the anthropologist Adrian Mayer working in Malabar in the 1940s (Mayer 1952: 150). An American-trained external observer reporting on communist rule in Kerala in the late 1950s evoked this wisdom of geopolitically-conscious Western demographers of the 1940s and 1950s. Commenting on Kerala as a state full of 'problems', he identified the root of all such (political) 'problems' to be economic, principally emanating from its 'overpopulation'. He wrote:

> The first impression that Kerala produces on the visitor is of a limited space overflowing with an almost limitless population. Kerala is itself a big village. No distinct villages exist but only a continuous line of hutments and habitations stretching almost roof to roof. Whatever centre we may take in Trivandrum, Kottayam, Ernakulam or Calicut, human beings seem to stretch out in all directions.… This lack of proportion between area and population is the main cause of Kerala's trouble. [Singh 1959: 12–13.]

This sordid picture, of a land bursting with unrest because too many people were pushing each other about, began to be endorsed within Kerala itself in the late 1950s:

> The unfortunate masses migrate from Kerala to other places due to inordinate increase in population and the centuries-old poverty have become a threat to the peaceful existence of India and the nearby States … if unemployment and poverty are rampant in Kerala, it is not given that other people must be made to suffer more than a fair share … Kerala's burning problems should be solved within Kerala itself. If birth control is not enforced by legislation, Kerala will continue to go from disaster to disaster whichever Golden Party may rule over it … [Nair 1958]

These voices grew shriller in the FPP propaganda of the 1960s. People who could not make a living in Kerala were projected as a potential political threat, or a possible source of shame for the Malayali people themselves within the Indian nation, as a visible symbol of our failure to develop. C.O. Karunakaran wrote: 'The terrible fires that raged in the slums of Madras is a meaningful danger-signal. Those who have no food and shelter will be ready to commit any extremity. They have nothing to lose.' Such starving masses are useless to the nation because they do not even pass health tests to become soldiers. 'It is these burgeoning third-rate people who pull the nation behind in not only national defense but also in all sorts of productive activities.' (Karunakaran 1967 b).

Kerala Kaumudi fully endorsed this:

> Already by now, Malayalis who suffer having no means for obtaining food, begging around for jobs and wandering through the other lands are the

laughing stock of others. We must give prominence to the Family Planning Programme if we are not to bear even greater insults and difficulties by bloating our numbers even further. [Editorial, *KK* 21 June 1967: 2.]

It was also as though individuals/individual states in national and global political systems were morally obliged to do whatever they could immediately, before asking for help, especially because the primary responsibility for creating such a sorry situation was forcefully laid upon them. Such beating-down of the sense of self-respect of Malayalis (as in the above quotes) could have had a considerable impact in 'norming' FP among the literate in Kerala. They were, of course, part of the Indian political system that resembled in many important ways the emergent post Second World War system of global governance that authorized the division of the world into formally equal nation-states, and made them formally responsible for their own material well being (Gupta 1999).

Obviously, this does not match very well with the understanding of poverty upheld by the then-hegemonic political force in Kerala, the communists, which was briefly mentioned earlier. But such opinions as this did not arouse much open protest. What was then the niche in which the FPP's claim to be the alleviator of poverty rested? I argue that it managed to escape, for most of the time, the hostile and critical scrutiny of leftist political society by choosing to base itself in apparently apolitical space: that of 'social uplift'. 'Social uplift'—or the conception of the 'social' as a domain in which the putatively apolitical work of 'uplifting' the poor and the weak took place—was familiar in the Malayali public sphere since the late nineteenth century through a variety of agencies. These included the missionaries, the state, and the community reform movements, and was widely pursued to be 'beyond politics'; a concern that bound all the different political opinions. It has been noted about the elaboration of the 'social' in nineteenth century north-western Europe that one of the striking effects of this 'social' was its dislocation of the political. The latter takes on an intensified air of privacy and invulnerability, of "high politics" associated with juridical and governmental power in a restricted manner. The question of poverty, for instance, becomes divorced from politics and assigned, especially in the work of the French political economists, to the social sphere. (Riley 1999: 51.) It has also been noted that this space was conceived of as eminently feminine—one in which the 'natural' qualities of the female sex could be put to good use (Riley 1999: 44–51). In Kerala too, the first generation of feminists tried very hard in the 1930s to claim the space of the 'social' as the legitimate space of feminine public activism (Devika 2006). These efforts were however hardly fruitful, and the 'social' remained pre-eminently a domain over which activisms stemming from community interests and the state made claims, which sometimes colluded and sometimes collided. Indeed, the 'social' has remained in Kerala a domain in and through which governmental power has vastly expanded, such that the more the former expanded, the more did the latter. The burden of a political history of the 'developmental phase' of Malayali modernity may lie in tracing the collusions and collisions of the 'political' and the 'social' as they expanded simultaneously in these times, and how subjects shuttled between these. Neo-Malthusianism in Kerala escaped critical scrutiny because of the neat bifurcation made between 'health reasons' (which E.M.S. Nambutiripad mentioned, cited earlier), found to rest in 'development,' and population control, a political issue. Thus, while the struggle over material resources came to be intensely politicized in Kerala in the mid-twentieth century, other forms of power and hierarchy continued to expand largely unsullied in 'social development'. Especially the form of élitism that privileged the 'cultured' over the 'uncultured', the decisive criteria of division being the values of the new modern educated élite.

Thus the FP propaganda identified its agents to be engaged in the ostensibly power-neutral task of 'uplifting' the inferiors and the ill-endowed. Its mien was one of noble self-sacrifice, required of the active agents of 'upliftment'. As in the case of the Christian missionaries of the nineteenth century, the entire life, energy, and material resources of this new variety of missionary too were to be devoted to the task of finally eliminating all that was below the line. Compliance of the (inevitably individual) objects of such 'upliftment' was to be secured not only by achievement of public endorsement but also by entering into their minds and thoughts. The lines of power were clearly laid out: the journey towards sameness could begin only when those who were below the line ceded all forms of resistance they could conceivably adopt and accepted the missionary as having superior knowledge and relied upon him/her as the guide towards a better life. This was characteristic of the earliest missionary interventions in Kerala, for instance in the well-known 'breast-cloth struggle' in southern Travancore in the nineteenth century, in which the missionaries supported the struggle of a lower-caste group, the Channars, against demeaning caste practices, and advanced their own moral agenda through it (Yesudasan 1975). It is striking how the latter made constant efforts to take control of the terms of the struggle; not that they were always and unambiguously successful (Jeffrey 1976).

To establish the inferiority of the targets of reform is an absolute necessity for missionaries. It is easier to make a people shorn of self-respect to accept charity, sympathy, and other forms of 'upliftment'; only such a people can be *acted upon*. Indeed, such acting–upon could be saturated with élitism, even when not advocating outright coercion. Justifying the prominence granted to sterilization in the FPP, an author wrote:

> Today, birth control is necessary for those in the lower ranks of society. These people have no thought of the future. Besides remaining steeped in superstition and evil customs, uncontrolled breeding as a solution for the troubles of life is spreading among them. Birth control is not even an issue for them. Only complete control will succeed among them. Therefore intensive propaganda about the important family planning technique of sterilization must be conducted among them and the male or female heads of all households with more than three children must be sterilized. [Ambady 1970.]

This statement does not directly demand forcible sterilization, but the élitist impatience with the 'overbreeding' masses, which authorizes urgent and intense, if physically non-violent intervention is difficult to miss. Secondly, while it indirectly admits to the existence of 'troubles of life' among the poor, this seems to require no solution. Only its effects are to be tackled, namely 'uncontrolled breeding', which is a nuisance to the state.

The task of 'uplift' being common to both the early developmental projects and missionary work, the connection between the ideal images of the FP worker and the missionary must not have been difficult to make. Writing about the rural development project at Marthandam in Travancore in the 1930s, Spencer Hatch remembered that the LMS missionaries working in the vicinity offered whole-hearted cooperation, saying that, 'This was needed to complete the Christian programme. When we had taught the people to live a better way of life ... many of them were actually too poor to live it' (Hatch 1932: 89). It is thus hardly surprising that developmental work seemed to be the natural extension of the missionary efforts to teach the people a 'better way' of life. The community development projects initiated in Travancore–Kochi in the early 1950s also drew upon the missionary-model in its early stages, and an early participant in these efforts has documented the missionary zeal of the development workers, who worked selflessly with the villagers, labouring to 'uplift' them, aiming at a non-violent revolution in the socio–economic life of the village (Rajasekharan 1991: 53–8). It is, then, hardly surprising that the FPP could have effectively accessed this pre-existing mode of drawing subjects. Whether or not general goals or aims converged, this specific path towards 'rural development' prescribed by the development-expert Spencer Hatch, succinctly described as 'Self-help with expert knowledge' (Hatch 1932: 6) seems to fit the FPP more than anything else, given its claim that reducing the numbers of individual families was the form of 'self-help' that could assist them most. As for expert knowledge, the crucial role that institutionalized expertise had in modern birth control was emphasized early enough. However, as to be expected within the missionary mode of creating subjects, tempering this 'expert' knowledge with intimacy was continually stressed. For persuasion to work, it was reminded, the FP agent was to get closely involved with the people, share their problems, clear up their doubts, allay their fears, assist them in all possible ways: in short, acquire the status of a friend and well-wisher.[22] If science had to be made more 'human', bureaucratic impersonality had to be avoided. As an author pointed out: 'It is everybody's duty to make ordinary people understand that harmless Family Planning methods are the products of scientific research and free of danger. If each person is not fired by an internal enthusiasm, the desired victory will not be attained.' (Kalyanikutty 1969: 5)

Thus the work of FP, it was often claimed, was not so much that of doctors and bureaucrats, but of those individuals and organizations that interacted intimately with the 'masses'. Thus a privileged role was conceded to voluntary organizations with a 'social uplift' or 'social service' agenda, ranging from élite gatherings like the Junior Chamber and the Lions Clubs to the humble women's associations and rural libraries.[23] The ideal FP worker would be fired by missionary zeal. Waxing eloquent on one such model worker, the *Matrubhumi* wrote:

> The weapon he uses to spread the message of Family Planning into the hearts of his 'patients' is music ... he has himself written a song carrying the message 'small family, happy family'. Whenever possible, he sings it to his 'patients' in a mellifluous voice ... Dr Mathew Thomas has undertaken Family Planning work with the zeal of a missionary. He has been able to muster the cooperation of his fellow-workers. In the Family Planning camp conducted in July, he and his colleagues bought a transistor radio as a prize for a lucky dip for acceptors. Imitating his model, another social worker of the area gifted a time-piece as second prize and the Panchayat contributed fifteen rupees as third prize ... Dr Mathew Thomas who practices the principles of Family Planning in his own life has but three children. [*Matrubhumi* 5 October 1966: 4.]

The FP worker's self-sacrifice combined with the brave struggle against superstition to shape an even-brighter halo around her/him. Condemning police brutality against picketing FP workers in Thrissur in 1969, the health minister of Kerala, B. Wellington, commented: 'The women who spread information regarding ways of preventing population increase in the countryside braving the suspicious and contemptuous glances of ordinary people in these times are performing a vital important duty to the nation. Giving them a raise of ten or fifteen rupees will only make country more prosperous; it will not ruin it.' (Varma 1969: 94.)

So while it was conceded that those officials and professionals who did not believe in the FPP were not to participate in it,[24] this could imply not just the liberal attitude of the state or its tolerance for dissenting views. Clearly, complete faith in the desirability of the FPP among the agents was identified as a key condition for its success. When such intentions were clear, then even the offering of cash incentives—which obviously went against the missionary project of 'mental conversion'—could be projected as justified. Hailing the architect of the successful Ernakulam mass sterilization camps, S. Krishna Kumar, as the ideal missionary–bureaucrat, the *Matrubhumi* argued precisely this. It pointed out that his motives were spotless, admitting that the popularity of the camps largely lay in the substantial sum being paid as incentive. This was however, 'neither inappropriate nor immoral. It is a practical tactic to make people ready to accept new ways of life instead of traditional beliefs' ('M' 1971). The incentives were often characterized as compensation for wages lost in the rest-period after surgery (for instance, Sadasivan 1970). The camp approach (or 'festival approach', as the FP publicists preferred to call it) was one designed to erect a temporary paradise free of inequalities and want. As a follow-up study on FP acceptors at the mass sterilization camp at Thiruvananthapuram expressed it:

> … It creates enthusiasm and a feeling of oneness and one purpose … Inside the camp all are advocates of birth control … The jubilant atmosphere, coupled with the generous and respectable treatment one gets, generates confidence, a purpose and a bright future. So the festival approach is appropriate and widely appreciated by the people. [Nair and Nair 1978: 9.]

However, this temporary paradise did not apparently last long, as if to set more oppressive realities in place. The above observers lamented that the problem with this approach was that promoters lack the missionary initiative, and seek only the incentives: 'Their interest lies in the number of sterilizations and not in the welfare of the person after the operation.' Another study conducted by the same authors showed that though only a week's rest was necessary to become fit for normal work after vasectomy, 'But here about 64% of the acceptors took more than thirty days to become fit for their normal work.... If this simple operation results in the loss of several weekdays and thereby the wages for the poor labourers, an unwillingness among them to undergo the operation is likely to develop.' (Nair and Nair 1978: 155). Such instances however certainly did not dissuade the FP publicists from attributing missionary righteousness to their cause.

Thus appearing completely shorn of all interest beyond altruistic 'upliftment', the FPP could well seem to be a radical force breaking down the authoritarian elements in the established 'traditional' order, while itself being committed to the building of a power-free society. No power was seen to be ensuing from dependence upon 'experts' and 'intimate counsel', sponsored by the state, the international aid agencies and the political powers of the first world. Such shortsightedness is best evident in the support given to artificial birth control, and to the FPP, by Ponkunnam Varkey, a leading figure among the Progressive writers. In Varkey's short stories (such as 'Anthony, Neeyum Acchanayoda?'), artificial birth control appeared as a radical taking-back of the reproductive capacities of individuals, freeing them from the clutches of an oppressive and exploitative Catholic Church. However, in the context of the FPP, this radical quality takes on a curious flavour. At the Ernakulam mass sterilization camp in 1971, Varkey stressed that those who dissuade ordinary people from accepting FP through 'propagating superstitions' are class enemies. He asked people 'not to be misled by the ideological confusions erected deliberately by a group of exploiters who have cornered all our resources' (*Matrubhumi* 20 July 1971: 2). The solution, however, does not even include, as one aspect at least, an effort to take back the resources thus unfairly concentrated. It exhorts the suffering and the exploited to adopt birth control, reduce their numbers, and by implication, end their sorrows through such 'self-help'. 'Class enemies', the nation, and the international geopolitics that drove FP initiatives in the third world at such a frenetic pace, all dissolve into the background. Besides, there were the others who felt that large families were the 'exploiters' as they allegedly consumed a greater share of the 'common pool' of resources (for instance, Justice M.U. Isaac, *Matrubhumi* 26 March 1968: 3).

The strategy of depoliticization was equally conspicuous in the FPP's approach towards the question of women's well-being and freedom. To a degree the FPP drew upon ideas that identified the social to be the place of women's public activism. We find innumerable statements that swear by the necessity to grant women a prominent role within the FPP both as agents and acceptors (for instance, *Malayalarajyam* 8 March 1956: 3; *MM* 6 January 1966: 5; *MM* 7 September 1960: 2; *KK* 11 August 1967: 2; editorial, *Matrubhumi* 7 January 1970: 4; *Matrubhumi* 19 November 1970: 7; *Matrubhumi* 28 November 1970: 4–5). Individual women and women's organizations were called upon to play an active part in the FP propaganda in the spirit of 'self-help' towards 'emancipation from biology', as that most ardent champion of FP, Dr S. Chandrasekhar, expressed it (*KK* 12 August 1969: 5). Incidentally, in the discourse of birth control, 'biological slavery' was identified early enough as something human beings ought to rebel against: Margaret Sanger made this point justifying birth control in the 1920s (cited in Dowbiggin 2002: 225). Many of the women who had been active in articulating the group-interests of 'Women' from the 1930s onwards were actively brought into the FP campaign, for instance Parvaty Ayyappan, Ambady Kartyayani Amma and T.C. Kochukutty Amma (*Matrubhumi* 25 July 1971: 2; *MM* 6 October 1960: 4; *Matrubhumi* 4 August 1966: 4). Yet, the practice of highlighting the victim-status of women as justification for interventions that sought to 'liberate' them was central to FP propaganda. Such rhetoric of 'liberation' assumed that passivity was a necessary correlate of women's oppressed condition: women oppressed by traditional family structures, therefore, were necessarily victims, passive sufferers, who could be rescued only through the active intervention of enlightened modern men (Devika 2007). Indeed, the stereotype of the victimized woman remained very much in the forefront of the FPP campaign both in the FPP propaganda, and in the writings of pro-FP authors. The woman oppressed by her biology was the symbol of the mass sterilization campaign at Ernakulam, and the architect of the campaign, S. Krishna Kumar, wrote:

> the symbol for this *Yajna* was an especially designed caricature—depicting a careworn and sad woman carrying on her hips an emaciated and undernourished infant and in her belly yet another child to be born—symbolising the desperate though latent demand of the mothers of the country for family limitation—and appealing silently to the world for Justice. [Kumar 1971: 36.]

The Malayalam movie, *Aswamedham* (1967) was praised for its realistic portrayal of the woes besetting the large family. Dr C.O. Karunakaran wrote about a particularly pathetic character in that movie:

> The heroine's mother dies at her tenth delivery. She had not borne it out of any desire on her part. That woman was sacrificed to the brutality of her leper-husband for whom *Guruvayoorappan* is the witness for everything. Three children died young. One contacted Leprosy. Death freed her from permanent hell. [Karunakaran 1967: 6.]

Here the reformer called upon to assume the role of liberator of the hapless women held in thrall by forbidding structures of tradition in early twentieth century Malayali reformisms assumes a new responsibility: to rescue the woman oppressed by her biology through sterilization. Needless to say, the non-reciprocity of relations implied in modern reformism came along with this. A poem published as part of FPP propaganda depicted a husband turning into an acceptor of FPP, moved by his wife's pangs of childbirth, her weakened state attributed to pregnancy, as if it were a pathology in itself (*Matrubhumi* 30 June 1970: 7). Sympathy was poured upon unfortunate wives whose cruel husbands refused to accept birth control, or allow them to do so. However, this did not seem to point to the solution of strengthening the position of women so that they could have a say in the matter. Faced with one such case, in which a woman whose philanderer husband refused to let her use contraception asked for some method she could practice without his knowledge, Dr C.O. Karunakaran could only 'sympathize'. Safer methods could only be adopted through common consent, and the pill was too expensive, and anyway, was only in the experimental stage. He lamented this sorry state, recommended even-more intensive FP propaganda, and the picketing of the unrelenting husband by FP workers and others as a last-ditch solution (Karunakaran 1970: 4). Yet the structures of domination within the family went completely unaddressed; indeed, the common agreement between this woman and the expert whom she approached for advice, that the existent structure should not be upset, seems to have been the very basis of the sympathy generated. While picketing seemed a valid-enough means to pressurize the husband into making a pro-FP decision, it scarcely raised the issue of the husband's control over his resisting wife's fertility. More glaringly, it ignored the conditions under which a woman's fertility became a burden to her. Almost paralleling Ponkunnam Varkey's speech cited above, here, the philanderer–husband was condemned as the very embodiment of patriarchal power that must be radically combated; but the 'radical fight' consisted not of efforts to unseat his authority, but was limited to the much milder measure of forcing him to accept FP. Also, while the visibility of the working of patriarchal power at the immediate level of the family was heightened, that of other, seemingly less immediate forms of control, as for instance, the manifold increase in the control exercised by the modern medical institution on women's bodies, was impaired. To mention another instance, a plea to end maternity leave and benefits to women workers with large families claimed that unemployed husbands impregnated their wives solely to claim such benefits. The solution to such powerlessness of women, however, was FP, and not any restructuring of family relations to give women a larger say (Pillai 1967).

In any case, most radical-sounding statements were more or less inevitably followed by the evocation of the duties of women–to be thrifty wives and responsible mothers. 'Emancipation from biology' seemed to be all the more committed to making women more efficient and hard-working agents in what was deemed their 'natural' domain, the home. The concern over women's health, so often voiced in the pro-FP and FPP propaganda literature inevitably issued the call for 'healthy mothers to manage healthy families', which in turn reinforced the thoroughly modern but no less burdening subject–position of the modern housewife deemed 'natural' to women. In the 1950s and '60s, the problems of working mothers balancing the responsibilities of the workplace and the home was frequently discussed,[25] and FP often came as a solution. Inevitably, the necessity of income from paid work by women outside the home was tied to the increasing material demands of the family. In debates over the advisability of women's paid work outside the home, those who supported it pointed out that it contributed to the financial security of the home, and the availability of contraception helped lighten domestic responsibility. Here again, FP is presented as an aid that enabled women to 'adjust' with some facility;[26] however, the entire issue of the double-burden of responsibility remained in limbo. We encounter exactly the same in the discussions about the efficacy of raising the age of marriage of women as a FP measure. There were various positions voiced on this question, but they were inevitably pivoted on whether or not such a measure would help to produce a woman capable of fulfilling the responsibilities of a housewife in a modern conjugal unit and household in both the physical and mental sense.[27] Those who argued for a lower age claimed that being impressionable will help the woman to fit with less friction into the new family as housewife; those who argued for a greater age claimed that the older the bride, the more mature she will be and better equipped to assume the responsibilities of housewife. At the same time, the 'lightening of the load' seemed, at best, ambiguous. Now women were expected to be evermore watchful mothers (their very adoption of FP was taken to testify that they were already so), to be increasingly responsible for the welfare of their (few) children—and prominent women in the Malayali public such as Leela Damodara Menon and Ambady Kartyayani Amma reminded their sisters about these responsibilities (*Matrubhumi* 19 November 1970: 7; *Matrubhumi* 4 August 1966: 4). Speaking at the half-yearly All-India Women's Conference meeting at Kochi in 1971, the Chief Minister of Kerala, C. Achyuta Menon, reminded women that gaining freedom must not mean abandoning 'their duties':

'Women must not forget their duties while seeking freedom.... In some countries where women have gained freedom children have been isolated from their parents. Do not deny children the love and affection of their parents ...' (*KK* 31 May 1971: 6). If physical labour was reduced, moral responsibility was doubled.

Thus 'emancipation from biology' certainly did not mean the liberation of women's reproductive capacities from the productivist modern family, or the channelling of women's energy into non-procreative concerns. There were, of course, exceptions like Dr O.K. Madhavi Amma who argued in favour of FP, that these were not times when women ought to devote all their time and energy to procreation and childcare (Amma 1971: 7). The rhetoric of the women's liberation movement in the West was sometimes drawn upon, as in a *Matrubhumi* editorial that strongly supported abortion, and argued in a recognizable feminist vein that women must control their reproductive capacities (2 June 1971: 4). However, whenever it seemed that there was a real prospect of women engaging in unregulated sexual activity, FP publicists immediately fell back, reiterating their commitment to 'safeguards' to maintain moral discipline—for instance, in strong opposition to a more liberal position on women's access to abortion (for instance *Matrubhumi* 5 January 1969: 7). Even when the direction of young girls exclusively towards marriage and family life was criticized, it was done in highly instrumentalist terms. A *Kerala Kaumudi* editorial commented: 'Our girls are keen on higher education. If employment for them is made plentiful then the tendency to think of marriage as the only way to live will die out.' This however is immediately attached to the imperative to control the growing population as an instrument; it was certainly not as a way of expanding the choices or life-options open to women (*KK* 7 January 1967: 2).

How deep the assumption regarding feminine nature, that it was 'naturally moral/ domestic', ran is amply illustrated in the following statement by Dr Kamala Ramaiyer, in an early speech answering common objections to FP. Flaying the claim that the ready availability of artificial contraception would lead women 'astray', she argued:

> But most women are dragged into evil ways not by the ready availability of facilities for artificial contraception. On the contrary, a close inspection would reveal that it is sheer poverty and the lack of the means to support children that lead women astray. [Ramaiyer 1959: 2.]

'Going astray' here probably refers to commercial sex. Here artificial contraception is tightly defined indeed, as 'family planning'. In its avatar as 'family planning', artificial contraception is the very safeguard of moral discipline, by virtue of its attributed capacity to fend off poverty. At the same time, it was sometimes argued that certain FP methods, particularly abortion, may promote laxity in self-discipline, and hence such services needed to be closely monitored. A divide between the essentially moral (i.e. perverted only in exceptional circumstances) and god-fearing rural women, and educated, well-off, possibly also urban women who are less so was also not infrequently posited. In a discussion about legalizing abortion conducted by the *Malayala Manorama* in 1970, Dr Mary John elaborated this point, claiming that rural women are not very likely to use this method, being quite god-fearing; however, 'One of the effects of legalizing abortions would be a greater demand for abortions from contraceptive-using educated women of prosperous families, who may seek these services upon becoming pregnant through the careless use of the instruments of birth control.' (*MM* 5 July 1970: I.) She, therefore cautioned that a vigilant system of monitoring be set up to regulate abortion services, to sort out the 'deserving cases'. Self-discipline emerges triumphant in either case; among poor women, it was to be reached by giving them access to FP services, whereas for well-off women, the reverse seemed to be required, i.e. a closely monitored and restricted access.

Some who wrote in these times sensed a general threat to the earlier project of individual self-building in the air, seeing it become increasingly a matter of governmental intervention and interest. As a prominent author remarked,

> today's new 'technique' is to apply external pressures upon human activities and instincts to make docile and control, in the same way as natural forces are tamed and controlled. This is political power itself—this path shapes the

duties and even the thoughts and emotions of each individual, making them dull and lifeless. [Menon 1969: 45.]

As for physical intimacy between men and women, the impatient rejection of fertility awareness-based contraceptive practices cancelled out the prospect of developing fertility control that would require an intimate awareness of each other's bodies by the sexual partners. The convenience of readymade non-procreative sex was to devalue the labour of love necessary for the latter. However, even such modern aspirations as these seemed to count little, not to mention non-modern sensibilities more or less shut out of public discussion as obsolete and superstitious. Indeed, clearly, Anthony Giddens' claims about the coming of 'plastic sexuality' through widespread contraception, with its promise of more democratic and non-instrumentalist sexual relationships (Giddens 1992) was miles away here.[28] Indeed, women seem to have been inserted all the more into a modernized regime of procreation, which was certainly as male-centred as the earlier ones. This was also fully in line with what the global pharmaceutical industries decreed: that women will remain the targets of contraceptive technology, though in many cultures men have traditionally taken a share of the responsibility in preventing pregnancies (Schneider and Schneider 1995). The development of male hormonal contraceptives, it seems, requires both a turnabout in the attitudes of the global pharmaceutical industry, and a renegotiation of masculine identities (Handelsmann 1991; Oudshoorn 2004).[29]

Notes

1 'Developmental idealism' was an outcome of a long and powerfully entrenched intellectual tradition originating from north-western Europe, which identified the societies there as the fullest fruition of human history, and hence the ultimate goal of all other societies in the world. It thus provided the criteria for evaluating other societies, and prescriptions for how these other societies might be transformed to resemble the West. Developmental idealism refers both to this faith and the various forms of activism that it entailed, which grew to enormous proportions under colonial conditions, and in post-colonial development in the third world. Arland Thornton,' The Developmental Paradigm, Reading History Sideways, and Family Change', *Demography,* 38, 4, 2001, 449–65.

[2] It involved, (1) freedom from major forms of social coercion and control stemming from the indigenous or traditional order, (2) the ability to chose rationally from among both indigenous and modern social, political, and cultural elements that seemed helpful in creating a productive, wealth-generating, disciplined new socio–economic order.

[3] The term 'new élites' may be preferable to 'middle-class' as it better indicates politico–cultural hegemony. Kunnathu Janardana Menon anticipated this when he identified the government servants, the graduates, the new rich, and the 'people' constituting a new *chaturvarnyam,* or caste system, in the place of the Brahmana, Kshatriya, Vaishya, and Shudra varnas. Menon, 'Abhinava Chaturvarnyam' (1934), in *Lekhavati,* Kozhikode, Prakashakaumudi Printing, 1955, 105–15.

[4] Another institution that aroused similar fears was cinema. See Bindu M. Menon, 'Shadow Lines: Cinema and Social Space in Early 20th century Thiruvithamkoor', paper presented at the SARAI Student Fellowship workshop, CSDS, New Delhi, 26 Aug. 2005.

[5] 'Santananiyantranam', *Rasikan,* 5, 5, 1934, 58–9.

[6] These points are made, more or less explicitly, in almost every piece of writing critical of birth control between the 1930s and 1950s that I have been able to see. A few may be cited here: P.M. Nair, 'Santananiyantranam' (Birth-control), *Arogyam* Special Issue, 1932, 76–9; 'Lokalokam' (Review of world affairs) in *Swajanaranjini* 1, 2, 1933–4, 33–41; 'Garbhaniyantranam' (Review of a book on artificial contraception), *Deepam,* 3, 5, 1932, 366; 'Santananiyantranam', *Aryan* 8, 5, 1935–6, 127–9; M.R. Madhava Warrier, Address to the Annual Conference of the Prakriti Vaidya Samajam (Association of natural healers), *Arogyam,* 2, 8/9, 1925–6, 41–56; 'Patradhipakurippukal' (Editor's notes), *Vanita Ratnam,* 7, 5/6, 1934, 133–4; 'Grihanayakan' (pseudonym), 'Aa Premeyam Jananániyantranamo Janannirodhanamo?' (What is that resolution: birth regulation or birth prevention?), *Nazrani Deepika* (henceforth, *ND*), 16 April 1951, 1–4; editorial, *ND,* 24 May, 1956; editorial, *Matrubhumi* 29 November 1952, 2; editorial, *Matrubhumi,* 27 Nov. 1955, 2; editorial, *Matrubhumi,* 1 Oct. 1952, 2; editorial, *Malayalarajyam* 19 Dec. 1959, 2; editorial, *ND* 2 Oct. 1960, 2; speech by Agamananda Swamikal, 7 March 1952, *Souvenir of the Fifteenth Haindava Mahasammelanam,* Haindava Sevaka Sangham, Thiruvananthapuram, 1952, 51–8. Several books and articles that use these arguments to build a critique of artificial birth control were also published during this period: see Amshi Narayana Pillai, *Mahatma Gandhiyude Atmasamyamanam* (Self-control as practiced by Mahatma Gandhi), Thiruvananthapuram, 1931–2; K.P. Kurup, *Vivaharangam* (The Arena of Marriage), Kozhikode, 1928; Ullattil Govindankutty Nair, 'Manushyavargathinte Bhaavi' (The future of humanity), *Vicharadhaara,* Kozhikode, P.K. Brothers, 1962, 24–36; Puthezhathu Raman Menon [1955], 'Laingika Pathanam' (Sex-education), in *Arivulla Ajnanikal,* Kottayam, SPSS, 1970, 11–17. Hostile

observers in the 1950s such as *Navasakti*, even saw a direct link between the comparatively free availability of the instruments of artificial contraception in these times to an alleged rise in adultery. Quoted in Venganoor Balakrishnan, *Balaramapuram G. Raman Pillai* (biography), Thiruvananthapuram, Navasakti Books, 2000, 100.

7 See report of Jayaprakash Narayan's criticism of the sterilization propaganda, *Matrubhumi*, 7 Nov. 1967; Editorial, *Malayala Manorama* (henceforth, *MM*), 9 July 1967, 2; *MM* 27 July 1961, 5. However, even in the 1980s, some commentators continued to claim that the widespread availability of reliable birth control methods had a negative effect on the sexual self-discipline of the youth. See E.A. Karunakaran Nair, 'Bhroonahatya Papamo?' (Is abortion a sin?), in *Buddhimanaya Putran Janikkan*, Kottayam, SPSS, 1984, 11–19.

8 See, also, Thomas Moonjoli,' Jananiyantrana Bhramam' (The folly of birth control), *ND* 4 June 1929, 5; J.J. Jacob, 'Santananiyantranamo' (Birth control?), *Nazrani Deepika* (*ND* from now), 17 June 1936, 8; Joseph Vitayathil, Speech in the Discussion on Motion no. 117, 30 July 1938, *Proceedings of the Travancore Sree Mulam Assembly*, vol. xii, part ii, 1939, 803.

9 'Santananiyantranam' (Birth control), *Aryakeralam* 1, 1, 1935–6, 5–6. Such arguments are also to be found in other 'humorous' writing, such as that of M.N. Govindan Nair. See 'Sadhukkal Bharttakkanmar' (Poor Husbands) [1936], in M.N. Govindan Nair, *Gopivilasam*, Kottayam, 1950, 50–6. For a 'serious' account much later, see P.T. Chacko, 'Kutumba Samvidhanam: Kutumbathinte Adiverukal' (Family planning: The roots of the family), *ND* 26 April 1959.

10 Speeches by Mrs I.C. Chacko and Anne Mascrene against artificial birth control at a protest meeting in Thiruvananthapuram, *ND*, 7 Jan. 1936, 4. Mrs I.C. Chacko is remembered as an outspoken champion of equal rights for women within the Syrian Christian community. See J. Devika, *Her-Self: Early Writings on Gender by Malayali Women*, Kolkata, Stree, 2005. Anne Mascrene was to be a well-known political figure, and an active presence in the struggle against the dewan's rule in Travancore. Also see, speech by the noted nationalist activist Ratnamayi Devi at the Nair Conference, *ND*, 15 April 1937, 7; speech by Annamma Kunjacko BABL at the All-Kerala Catholic Congress, *ND* 12 April 1950, 1; speech by Mariakkutty John BABL at the All-Kerala Catholic Congress, *ND* 15 May 1951, 2; speech by Mrs Malloor Govinda Pillai at the Nair Conference, *Malayala Rajyam*, 18 Nov. 1953.

11 See, for instance, P.T. Chacko, 'Kritrimasantananiyantranam' (Artificial contraception), *Deepika Weekly*, 5, 8, 1952, 3–10; Louis Mathias, 'Santananiyantranam', *Deepika Weekly*, 4, 1, 1951, 16–20; editorial, *ND* 3 Dec. 1935, 3; 'Nireekshakan' (pseudonym),' 'Santananiyantranam: Atu Sweekaryamano?' (Birth control: is it acceptable?), *ND*, 7 Jan. 1936, 1; editorial, *ND*, 15 April 1958, 2; 'M', 'Kritrimasantananiyantranam Streetvathinu Orapamanam' (Artificial contraception: an insult to womanhood), *ND*, 2 Oct. 1960, 5.

[12] *Mahila,* commenting on *Kesari*'s suggestion that women legislators should petition the government to initiate family planning measures in Travancore, wrote: 'Is the notoriety of being 'deniers of Motherhood' an ornament to the women of Travancore? Surprising!' ('Mahilabhashanam', *Mahila,* 11, 10, 1931, 5). However, in 1932 this position changed, now claiming that birth control was a necessity in Travancore and hinting that women ought to pay attention to this. See 'Janasankhya Vardhippikkano?' (Should population be increased) in 'Mahilabhashanam', *Mahila,* 12, 1, 1932, 160–1.

[13] See, for example, editorial, *ND,* 29 Dec. 1956, 2; report of speech by Joseph Pettah, *ND,* 21 Jan. 1936, 1; M.O. Joseph, 'Jananniyantranaprasthanam' (The birth control movement), *ND,* 22 Dec. 1933, 8.

[14] See, for instance, M.R. Velupillai Sastry, *Purogamanasahitya 'Kolahalam'* (The 'furore' over progressive literature), Thiruvananthapuram,Educational Supplies Depot, 1948, 150–4; Narikkuzhi, *Kutumbathinu Nere* (Against the family) (pamphlet)) Aluva, S.H. League 1954 (1952); Brother Vadakkan, 'Sa. Damodaran Sannadhanano?' (Is Comrade Damodaran ready?), *Tozhilali,* 26 July 1953, 8; George Nellayi, 'Communist Vyavastayil Kutumbe Bhadrataikkulla Sthanam' (The place of family stability within the communist system), *Deepika Weekly,* 5, 27, 1952, 16–17; T.J. Job, 'Russiayum Sadacharavum' (Russia and morality), *Deepika Weekly,* 5, 13, 1952, 23–25; Speech by Annamma Chacko Kalarickal at the Knanaya Catholic Congress, *ND,* 22 May 1960, 2; editorial , 'Samaram Arambhichateyullu' (The struggle has just begun), *Navasakti,* 5 Aug. 1959, cited in Venganoor Balakrishnan, *Balaramapuram G. Raman Pillai* (biography). Thiruvananthapuram, Navasakti Books, 2000, 198.

[15] By the ideology of modern gender I mean: (a) the presupposition of the division of the world into 'public' and 'domestic' domains, appropriate for men and women respectively, to which they are to remain committed for life, (b) compulsory heterosexism, (c) a strong claim to represent the 'natural' foundations of the human social order, with the cautionary rider that for this 'natural' aspect of humanity to manifest in society, a great deal of social activity, ranging from legal interventions to training through modern education, is necessary.

[16] This is well-illustrated in V.T's writings: the sexually active heroines he constructs in his short stories may be contrasted to the sordid picture of Umadevi Naripetta, in V.T. Bhattatiripad *Karmavipakam* (autobiography), Changanashery, Best Books, 1988, 284–96, whose active sexual desire did not remain subservient to the interests of the community.

[17] Indeed, it has been pointed out that the modernists in the West manifested a similar ambivalence about the issue of birth control, and that this reveals that the modernist ambition to break away from realism's evolutionary narrative was never fully successful. See Christina Hauck, 'Abortion and the Individual Talent', *ELH,* 70, 1, 2003, 223–66. Also, the suggestion that categories such as 'realists' and 'modernists' are far from objective evaluations, and therefore a more objective assessment of these 'is to deprivilege them as literature, treating each

instead as discourse, subject to the same rules and constraints as any other discourse' (Astradur Eysteinsson, *The Concept of Modernism,* Cornell, Cornell University Press, 1990, 183–4) seems also fully relevant for the categories in modern Malayalam literature.

18 Some of these articles were: Paravur K. Gopala Pillai, 'Chila Dambatyasastra Rahasyangal' (Some secrets of conjugal science), *Kutumbapatrika,* 2, 2, 1934,10–12; Speech by Dr G.H. Gray at the auspices of the YMCA, *Kutumbapatrika,* 2, 4, 1934, 4; 'M.S.' (pseudonym) 'Kutumbajeevitam', *Malayala Manorama Weekly,* 50, 20, Nov. 1948, 19–22. To mention some of the books: *Lingavijnanam: Balabodhini,* (Sex education for boys) Thrissur, Gandhi Grandhalayam, 1955; *Lingavijnanam: Balikabodhini* (Sex education for girls), Thrissur, Gandhi Grandhalayam, 1955; *Purushanmarude Laingikaroganagal* (Sexual diseases of men) Thrissur, Gandhi Grandhalayam, 1955; E.A. Karunakaran Nair,'*Njan Engane Undayi*? (How was I Born?), Kottayam, SPSS, 1968; P.M. Mathew, *Ningalude Jeevita Prasnangal* (Problems in Your Life), Kottayam, 1968; Punalur Sudarshanan Nair, *Premavum Dambatyavum* (Love and Marriage), Kottayam,1970; V.R. Menon, *Ina Cherumbol* (While Mating), Thrissur, Mangalodayam, 1970.

19 Popular magazines of the 1950s and 1960s, such as *Kaumudi*, *Malayalarajyam*, *Malayala Manorama Weekly,* and others published a great many articles on human psychology precisely in this spirit. For instance, see, K. Kuttappan, 'Kuttikalude Anveshanabuddhi' (The inquisitiveness of children), *Malayalarajyam Weekly,* 12 Dec. 1965, 16–18; K.G. Kesavan Nair, 'Manasinte Atbudhasaktikal' (The wondrous powers of the mind), serialized in *Malayalarajyam Weekly*, Oct.—Nov. 1956. *Malayala Manorama Weekly* used to run a regular column on psychology written by V.K. Alexander. See 'Akarana Bhayam' (Unreasonable fear), *MM Weekly,* 50, 2, 29 Aug. 1948, 25–6. A prominent author writing on human psychology was Vakkom M. Abdul Khadar whose articles published in the 1940s have been collected in *Vicharavedi*, Punalur, Udaya Publishing, 1947. These magazines constituted an important resource through which modern psychology began to draw its subjects; the psychology column in *MM Weekly* promised to answer its readers' queries. *MM Weekly* 50, 9, 17 Oct. 1948, 15–16. They also served to assert the relevance of modern psychology to other fields such as, for example, pedagogy. See V.V. Abraham, 'Adhyapakanmarum Manassastravum' (Teachers and psychology), *MM Weekly,* 50, 11, 31 Oct. 1948, 14–16.

20 See Viji Velappan, 'Santushta Kutumbam: Adyam Tanne Adittara Paniyuka (The happy family: build the foundation first), *MM,* 12 June 1970, 6; Mrinalini, 'Kalyanam Kaliyalla' (Marriage is no play) *Matrubhumi Weekly,* 41, 10, 26 May 1963, 28; Padmini Balakrishnan, 'Kutumbajeevitam Enthinu? Engane?' (Family life: for what? How?), *Matrubhumi Weekly,* 41, 16, 7 July 1963, 29; Sati Ramachandran, 'Udyogastakalaya Matakkalum Kunhungalum' (Working mothers and children), *KK,* 4 May 1970, 5; C.K. Lilly, 'Bharyayaya Udyogasta' (The working woman who is also a wife), *KK,* 3 March 1968, 4; V. Subhadra

Devi, 'Bharyayaya Udyogastaye Patti' (A reply to C.K. Lilly), *KK,* 10 March 1968, 6. All these issues and arguments are humorously engaged with in the 'Kunji' series written by the popular humourist of these times, P.K. Rajaraja Varma, whose heroine Kunji is the barely-educated wife of a lawyer, Panju Menon, negotiating with what gets presented to her as 'modernity'. See for instance, his *Kunjiyammayude Chintakal*, Calcutta, Rashmi Publications, 1969, 60–104.

21 This does not however really mean that all communists adopted an unambiguous anti-birth control position. Indeed not. Some of the fellow travellers of the communists were ardent propagandists of FP, such as V.R. Krishna Aiyer and Dr A R. Menon. See, for instance, speeches by Dr A.R. Menon and Thoppil Bhaskaran Pillai, Discussion on Demands for Grants: Medical, Public Health and Capital Outlay on Public Health, 20 March 1959, *Proceedings of the Kerala Legislative Assembly,* vol. vii, 1960: 2000–3; speech by V.R. Krishna Aiyer, Discussion on Demand for Grants: Medical, 19 June1957, *Proceedings of the Kerala Legislative Assembly,* vol. i, 1958, 1498–1502.

22 For excellent instances of such argument, see, G. Velayudhan, 'Enthanee Kutumbasamvidhanam' (What is this FP), *KK,* 24 Sep. 1967, 5; 'Sanatananiyantranam Arkkuvendi?' (Birth control for whom?), *KK,* 29 March 1970, 3; K. Narayana Aiyar, 'Balaramapuram Camp', *KK,* 15 May 1968, 3–4. There were also explicit criticisms of the bureaucratization of FP. See, *Malayalarajyam,* 13 Sept. 1964, 5.

23 Innumerable speeches and articles on this theme carry this exhortation. For a few, see speech by Dr S. Chandrasekhar to the Bharat Sevak Samaj, reported in *Matrubhumi,* 2 Oct. 1968, 6; report of inaugural speech by the health minister of Kerala, B. Wellington, at FP Seminar at Thiruvananthapuram in *KK,* 26 April 1968, 8; editorial, *KK,* 12 July 1970, 2. Voluntary organizations such as the Bharat Sevak Samaj, business clubs committed to social service such as the Lions' Club, the Rotary Club and the Junior Chamber were actively involved in organizing and funding camps; so also were *mahila samajams.* One important reason identified for the success of the Erankulam camps was the enthusiastic participation of the voluntary organizations. See Grace Kurien, 'Ernakulatte Kutumbasootrana Camp Oru Mahatbhutam' (The Ernakulam camps: a great miracle), *Matrubhumi,* 25 July 1971, 4.

24 See answer to starred question by P.C. Raghavan to Home Minister P.C. Chacko, 22 July 1960, Second Session, *Proceedings of the Kerala State Legislative Assembly,* vol. 1961, 2447–49; statement by health minister in the Kerala Legislative Assembly that Catholics and other doctors with conscientious objections to sterilization would be exempt from such duties. First Session, 19 Jan. 1968, *Proceedings of the Kerala State Legislative Assembly,* vol. xxii, 1969, 615–19.

25 For some articles that raise these issues, see Soma Krishna Pillai, 'Veetammamar Vazhittiruvil' (Housewives at crossroads), *MM,* 10 Oct. 1969, 6; Dhanya Narayanan, 'Kutumbam Innale, Innu, Nale' (The family: yesterday, today,

tomorrow), *MM,* 19 Sept. 1969, 6; Subaida Beevi, 'Udyogasthayaya Matavu Kutumbattinu Shapamo?' (The officer-mother: a curse to the family?), *MM,* 23 Oct. 1969, 7; Lalita Mohana Panikker, 'Streekalkku Oru Putiya Veekshanam Avashyam' (Women need a new vision), *KK,* 16 March 1969, 4; Annamma Jacob, 'Udyogastayaya Kutumbini' (The employed housewife), *MM* 22 Oct. 1971, 6; V. Subhadra Devi, 'Bharyayaya Udyogastaye Patti' (About the employed wife), *KK,* 10 March 1969, 6.

[26] See Usha Sukumaran, 'Udyogastayaya Bharya: Oru Vishadeekaranam' (The employed wife: an explanation), *MM,* 19 Nov. 1971, 3; Gracy Cheriyan, 'Akattum Purattum Modiyulla Veedu' (A house splendid inside and outside), *MM,* 27 Nov. 1970, 6; Annamma Kurian, 'Jananniyantranavum Kutumbinikalum' (Birth control and housewives), *MM,* 28 Nov. 1969, 6; Annamma Joseph, 'Bharya Udyogastayayal' (When the wife is employed), *MM,* 6 July 1969, 4.

[27] See the discussion in the 'Yuvakkal Chintikkunnu' column of *Matrubhumi,* 14 July 1968, 4; 21 July 1968: 4; see also the discussion on the same topic in the *MM*, in *MM,* Sunday Supplement, 21 Aug. 1970, 6; *MM,* 4 Sept. 1970, 6. See also, C.K. Lakshmikutty Amma, 'Janaperuppavum Vivahaprayavum' (Population increase and the age of marriage), *Malayalarajyam,* 26 Aug. 1967, 3.

[28] However, as the recent literature reveals, FP need not always have such consequences as these: indeed, it can lead to the decoupling of sexuality from both biological and social reproduction in non-Western societies too. Daniel Smith argues this point in his work on the Igbo of Nigeria. However, this, again, does not mean that Western values have been accepted, and local ones rejected wholesale. See, Daniel Jordan Smith, 'These Girls Today *Na War-O*: Premarital Sexuality and Modern Identity in Southeastern Nigeria', *Africa Today,* 47, 3/4, 2000, 99–120.

[29] It may also be added that the population control establishment was too obsessed with creating 'simple methods', eventually seeking to replace women's control of contraception with governmental and medical control of population growth in the definition of 'use-effectiveness'. See Marcia L. Meldrum, '"Simple Methods" and "Determined Contraceptors": The Statistical Evaluation of Fertility Control 1957–1968', *Bulletin of the History of Medicine,* 70, 2, 1996, 266–95.

2

Domestication, Family Happiness and Family Planning

Child-Crafting and the Modern State

The dominant literature on Kerala's demographic transition is clear about the reasons for the widespread adoption of the small family norm. The explanation offered is often twofold. First, the economic conditions under which the costs of bringing up children increased manifold is pointed to (but the implications of this observation are rarely developed) (Panikar et al. 1984; Zachariah 1984; Mahadevan and Sumangala 1987; Stein 1995; Padmadas 2000). And secondly, the far-reaching changes in twentieth-century Malayali society are presented as releasing progressive forces that 'liberate' the individual, such that the small family norm appears as something that a progressive society would automatically gravitate towards (Ramachandran 1997: 205–356). That the adoption of the small family norm has not significantly widened the range of life-options available to women, or made child-rearing less anxiety-ridden, is easily overlooked.

In this chapter I intend to examine how modern familial arrangements proposed in the mid–late nineteenth century, and increasingly actualized in the twentieth, played a decisive role in directing Malayalis towards state-sponsored contraception. These were important in facilitating the state's intervention in the domestic domain, which later enabled it to play an active role in the FP campaign without arousing much resistance. This is related to, but distinct from, the casting of the ideal of the sexually disciplined individual discussed in the former chapter. In other words, here I wish to explore how Malayalis were drawn into the discourse of FP as 'responsible householders/home managers'. Secondly, I make a few tentative suggestions regarding the shaping of material circumstances in which the new ideal of the small family appeared not only desirable, but also vital for survival, for diversely-located sections of people. That, gender strongly mediated these processes will probably be evident in the course of this chapter. This may help us garner some insights into why contraception in Kerala is an instrument that bound together the new patriarchal family, and not one that threatened it, notwithstanding claims here of women's 'greater enlightenment'. Besides, it may, later, lead us to a critical discussion about the varieties of anxieties that have accumulated around the small family in contemporary Kerala, as expressed in the media, literature, cinema, religious and medical discourses.

There seems to be some reason to question the long-naturalized association between the idea of the modern family and the small family norm in Kerala. First, even a cursory survey of the FP propaganda literature of mid-twentieth century Kerala would convince one of the massive efforts to link the two. One is struck by the sheer number of words spent on 'positively' linking this association. That is, in arguing that the possibilities offered by the nuclear family are best realized when the number of children is kept low. Secondly, examining early reformist demands for change in the family form and the reformist critical appraisals of the joint family, there is little that links the desired ideal of the modern family (constituted by two major axes, the husband–wife and parents–children, supported economically by the self-earned income principally of the father, and managed by the mother) to the small family norm. Indeed, in some of the early defences of patriliny in which the nuclear family figures as the 'natural' and sole possible outcome of the adoption of patriliny, the possibility of raising large families is counted as one of the key advantages (for instance, Mathen [1865] 1993). Thirdly, it may be possible to argue that modern domesticity, as projected in early and mid-twentieth century Malayali society, could well be read as implying a system quite conducive to bringing into being more children than less. The conception of marriage as an unambiguous lifelong association; the identification of a 'natural' provider of economic sustenance with total and personal responsibility for it; the incitement and direction of fresh energies in women towards the constant monitoring of children, all support such a claim. Lastly, there were strong countervailing pressures such as furiously competitive community politics since the early twentieth century (Ouwerkerk 1994; Menon 1994; Mammen 1981), which may have implied the promotion of the large, rather than small, family. However, that the small family norm eventually triumphed alerts us to the need to provide historical understanding of this triumph. The last question needs to be explored in some detail: why was it that neither frenetic community politics nor the evocation of 'United Kerala' in mid-twentieth century led to the questioning of population reduction. Malayali national interest, it seemed, was poised upon the reduction of the number of Malayalis, and not on their increase.

One way to begin this inquiry is to look for elements within the ideal of the modern family propagated in the early twentieth century Malayali society that might have suited the small family norm. Here the significance of the attribution of personal responsibility to the parents (in a uniquely gendered fashion, of course) emerges. In projections of modern domesticity, the agencies of the father/ householder and the mother/home manager were constructed in a way that the state could appeal directly to them, overlooking intervening institutions such as the locality, the extended family, or community. Nevertheless, the opening up of agencies within the domestic domain that the state could easily access cannot alone explain why the small family norm became such an integral part of the ideal of modern family in Malayali society. There was a certain conjunction of discursive and non-discursive factors, quite apart from the state's promotional efforts, that made small family size appear an inevitable element of the ideal modern family. Prominently, the process by which a certain notion of family subsistence as basically involving scarce means and unending wants gained ground steadily and substantially among different social groups requires serious attention here. A full-scale attempt to map out the different routes and temporalities by which differently situated and endowed groups may have arrived at such a notion is well beyond this chapter. Here I shall endeavour only to make some preliminary forays.

Above all, my intention is to bring to light the political content of what has been largely recognized as a 'social process'; the gradual sedimentation of the small family norm. In the first place, I contend that a process of 'domestication' has been one of the major processes of social change emergent in Malayali modernity. Both the senses of the term are important here. I claim that the small family norm and the consequent preference for family limitation is part of a process in and through which people have been directed towards investing most of their time, energies, and desires in the home. At the same time, this also implies a certain 'taming', a making useful, a political docility, of individuals. Nancy Folbre's notion of 'child-crafting' seems relevant here (Folbre 1998). The more the domestic domain became a space for shaping perfect individuals, the more child-rearing has resembled a craft-like activity in which children are treated as a form of 'raw material' upon which parents work. This offers the parents a tantalizing mix of emotional intensities, pleasure, and pain. Parenting is then persistent, even agonizing, labour, combined with the pleasure of near-total absorption and insulation from any larger worries stemming beyond the home, and the pleasurable, if precarious, expectation of a perfect end-product. The strains and tensions of domestic responsibilities and its pleasures and consolations all stem from a common source: the direction of a major share of the energies of men and women into their supposedly natural calling, parenting. This undoubtedly has important implications for the 'public action' recognized as a major force that drove the 'Kerala Model' (Parayil 2000), and for the history of citizenship in modern Kerala. It may be possible to claim that family planning both benefited from and accelerated this process of 'domestication'.

Secondly, I contend that we need to question the literature on Kerala's achievements in improving human life, which have largely tended to treat the processes leading to such achievements as power-free. Noteworthy efforts to recognize the importance of institutional change in bringing about fertility decline have often taken this line. For instance, Monica Das Gupta (1999) has argued that the shift towards fewer number of children 'is related to cognitive changes wrought by the replacement of deeply hierarchical socio–political institutions by the more egalitarian institutions of modern governance' (p. 1). She draws upon the familiar account of the combined effect of widespread education, better health care, and the loosening of traditional institutions (p. 6) to explain the fertility transition in Kerala. While there is no doubt that the death rate has fallen and the general health of the population improved, the assumption that these processes were insulated from power-regimes seems somewhat naïve. Modern power, as Michel Foucault has so powerfully shown, does not banish pleasure, nor is it principally hinged upon the taking of life. Rather, it fosters life. In the rooting of what Foucault calls 'bio-power' (Foucault 1978: 138–9)—the two poles of which are the 'anatomo-politics of the body' and the 'bio-politics of population'—in Malayali society, the family has been a major focus. The family has served as the vehicle of both these forms of regulation, and the success of the latter seems to have been crucially dependent on the effective rooting of the former. Pursuing the history of Kerala's social development in this fashion, the possibility of viewing the success of family planning in mid-twentieth century Kerala as a *political* event—involving the entrenchment of new networks of power—is unfurled. Indeed, scholarship on the dissemination of FP elsewhere too have stressed the degree to which it has generated new effects of power, especially in non-Western societies (for instance, Newland 2001). Indeed, I find Greenhalgh's (1990) suggestion more compelling not only because it eschews universal explanations, but also because it is sensitive to questions of inequality: 'fertility transitions may best be construed as products of change in class-specific opportunity structures in response to transformations of global and regional economies ... the adoption of contraception may be an eminently political process, both reflecting and exacerbating power differentials between the sexes and class' (p. 98).

The Impossibility of Carefree Breeding

From the latter half of the nineteenth century, we increasingly encounter in writings, the determined articulation of a notion of 'responsible parenting', which gained nearly unchallenged acceptance among the educated social groups in mid-twentieth century Malayali society. This attributed to parents the complete, personal, and 'natural' responsibility for the well-being of children. It also implied the loosening of the ties of men, women, and children with larger kin groups, the locality, or the community, and fashioned them as husbands, wives, and their children within a single unified institution, recognized as the modern family. Further, it prominently foregrounded a gendered division of domestic responsibility ostensibly grounded in the difference in the 'natural' sexual endowments of bodies. In the modern family, the father was to be the chief provider of economic support, while the mother was to manage the materials and souls within the domain of the domestic. The activity of parenting was ideally projected to be a sort of child-crafting, in which the parents sought to mould their offspring into full-fledged individuals.

It is not difficult to see that this must have been quite a novel suggestion. Accounts of the upbringing of the young from late nineteenth and early twentieth century society gleaned from autobiographies (and from the accounts of anthropologists working here much later) seem to confirm its novelty. The division of labour involved in the socialization of the young appears to have been far more spread-out over different agents, including elders and senior kin in the extended family, and retainers and servants in the case of well-off joint families. (Rao 1957; Nambutiripad 1963; Kesavan 1965; Menon 1971; Kunhappa 1981). From within this complicated network with its multiple levels and hierarchies, complex and mobile relations of domination and resistance, the husband and wife along with their children were to be culled out and re-established as a self-sufficient unit unto itself. The new unit was to turn around two major axes. One was the husband–wife axis, which was seen to be constituted by mutual bonding in moral obligations, mutual moral shaping, romantic love, and the wife's obligation to provide aesthetic pleasure (Devika 2007). The second axis of the modern family was to be the parent–child relationship. This was seen to be constituted by the bonding effected through, first the supposedly 'natural' affinity and affection of the parents towards their children, and secondly by a social obligation to mould them into fully individualized adults. With these two axes in place, the modern family was expected to function as an efficient institution for the production of industrious, rational, and self-disciplined subjects, with the husband and wife playing their respective gender-ordained roles, complementing each other's contribution.

These were also times in which pleas were begun to be made on behalf of a new, all-encompassing collectivity, the Nation. Travancore, Cochin or the projected Indian nation of the future most often occupied this space. Such pleas urged people to improve their agriculture by adopting new techniques and working harder to produce for the market, embrace profit-oriented industrial production for a wider market, and directed them to various wealth-generating activities (for instance, Varma 1874). It also seemed that the other requirement to enter the promised land of material prosperity and temporal power, enticingly mirrored in the nations of Europe and North America, was to persuade parents to fulfil their 'natural responsibilities' towards children, so that subjects capable of wealth-production would be produced. Another backdrop against which such role-assumption appeared vital was the articulation of a vision of a society of equals capable of completely erasing the hierarchies prevalent within the established social order(s), which privileged *janmabhedam* or difference by birth. In these projections of such an ideal social order, human beings were valued not by the 'purity of their blood' or by caste, but by the weight of their individual qualities alone. Thus, in such a society, gender alone, appearing to be 'naturally given', was taken to be the only enduring social division. Accompanying such projections were pleas for correct training to sharpen internalities through proper upbringing and education of the young to hasten the downfall of the *janmabhedam*–determined social order(s) and actualize the vision of the society of equals. Among the institutions identified as areas for such training, the modern family occupied a prime position (Devika 2007). Thus it is no coincidence that throughout the period from late nineteenth century up to the present, concerns about social and individual discipline in Malayali society have inevitably gravitated towards the state of the modern family. In this, nineteenth century Protestant missionaries, modernizing state officials, twentieth century women's associations, community movements, social reformers, nationalists, communists, late-modern religious cult-followers, the Catholic Church, demographers, educationists and economists, psychologists and family counsellors, not to speak of the institutions of law and order, have found common ground.

The task of shaping the modern patrilineal family turning upon the husband–wife and parents–children axes was found to be especially pressing in Malayali society in which a significant section of the people lived within matrilineal domestic arrangements, too often berated as hideous and 'unnatural' in Victorian reckoning (for instance, in the writings of the prominent missionary, Augusta Blandford, Blandford 1904). Nor did a local model seem readily available for imitation. The practice of patriliny among the Syrian Christians or among the Malayala brahmins seemed quite distant from the ideal model imported from north-western Europe. Even those who did not savour imported models sought other similar models closer home, like the family life of the Tamil brahmins (Nambutiripad 1925). And even for those who were reluctant to swallow the missionary representation of the existent marital arrangements, like O. Chandu Menon, the standard of reference was still the monogamous family with the lifelong union of husband and wife (Kodoth 2001).

Making men accept the role of the chief provider of their wives and children was, not surprisingly, often identified as the first step towards the setting up of the modern family. The criticism mounted against matriliny by the CMS missionary George Mathen illustrates the shape of the arguments that not only survived many generations but were also accentuated and intensely moulded in and through each of them. Entrusting the father and mother with the responsibility for the well-being of their children seemed the surest way of ensuring the longevity of the monogamous marital bond, the absence of which seemed to underlie a 'decline' of Nairs. In return, the enduring husband–wife relation was seen to produce superior progeny:

> As, in current practice, the authority over guardianship lie in the uncles, the fathers have no interest and responsibilities in their affairs. In contrast, if patriliny were the rule, fathers would have had concern for the care and wellbeing of their offspring, and would not abandon the mothers of their children. Because of this difference, the mothers too would not reject the husbands of their youth, and seek after other men.... Children born to couples living in mutual fidelity are found strong and healthy, but the offspring of those who lead a loose and stray life are mostly weak and sickly. [Mathen [1865] 1993: 351.]

Mathen claims that matriliny, originating under primitive conditions lacking in religion, ruled out the possibility of 'natural parental love' in fathers, as they could not recognize their progeny (p. 348). Moving towards the 'natural', to him, seemed to call for the constitution of the patrilineal monogamous family in which a strict division of labour between father/ householder and mother/ homemaker was already in place. Human infants, it was pointed out, unlike animals, required

> not only food but also clothes to wear and training in some trade. Since they have neither the capacity nor the time to labour during the training, they have to be fully provided for in this period with not only food and clothes but also the entire expenses of education. Since the mother lacks the capacity to create the wealth necessary for this, the father's help is most essential. But if fathers have no authority over children and can expect no favour from them later, they will show little interest ... [Mathen [1865] 1993: 351–2]

Therefore although the parental love of the father springs 'naturally', some cultural manipulation appears to necessary for it to concretize: the occupation of the seat of paternal authority over the children by the father seems to be a precondition for such love to blossom. Innumerable reformist texts seeking to establish an economic base upon which to build the modern family would reiterate precisely this combination of nature and culture. Bonds of affection between uncles and nephews and nieces were judged not entirely natural and therefore not sufficiently 'basic'. The lack of 'love' in matrilineal joint families was often lamented by Nair reformers, and ascribed to the 'unnatural' familial arrangements prevalent (for instance in the autobiography of the Nair reformer Mannath Padmanabha Pillai, in Pillai 1977). Notwithstanding these claims, we do have other autobiographical accounts in which the uncle–nephew bond appears no less intense and affectionate than that between father and son (for instance, Menon 1959).[1] Educated Nairs became avid supporters of the theory that the father making provision for his children was simply following the 'dictate of natural law', at the turn of the nineteenth century. This is evident in their responses to the queries of the Malabar Marriage Commission (see *Report of the Malabar Marriage Commission* 1891: 171), and in the speeches by early Nair reformers like Sir C. Sankaran Nair (*Malayala Manorama* 11 June 1910). By the twentieth century, the idea that a man's labour and wealth were to be utilized for the well-being of his immediate family gained rapid strides. The report of the Ezhava Law Committee of Travancore actually claimed in 1919 that the practice of marriage of the Ezhavas of Travancore was actually very close to the modern patrilineal monogamous model. It emphasized that the community was in favour of a law enjoining strict monogamy, and that this type of marriage was both 'natural' and 'conforming to the line and tendency of civilization', and that in most cases 'the Ezhava wife lives with her husband and under his protection' (*Report of the Ezhava Law Committee* 1919: 9). Any other suggestion would, increasingly, seem unfair or impractical. During the tour of the Ezhava Law Committee, a member of the committee is said to have asked Sree Narayana Guru, one of the foremost spiritual and reformist figures in Kerala, who the rightful heir of a man's self-earned wealth was. He apparently replied that the dead man's neighbours were his true heirs. The compiler of this anecdote records that the suggestion was immediately dismissed as 'impractical' (quoted from Mooloor S. Padmanabha Panikar's memoirs in Bhaskaran 2000: 238).[2]

The actualization of the role of the father/householder was deemed important by some seekers of reform of modern education, as it developed in early twentieth century Malayali society. One such instance was the proposal put forth by L.A Ravi Varma Tampuran in 1924–25, which devised a special subject called *Grihastadharmam* (Householder's Duties) for boys, which was to comprise 'Methods of producing and utilizing wealth, obligations and duties towards parents, spouse and children, and the world in general, principles of the correct instruction of the young. Through this subject the pupil may be made fairly well aware of his duty.' (Tampuran 1924–25: 220). Such concerns about transforming men into responsible householders attained considerable visibility in the agendas of virtually all community movements. The image of the modern (read wealthy, prosperous, politically powerful) community, when projected in the speech and writing produced from within community-movements, seemed to consist of several such disciplined and productive families coming together. This was a perennial theme surfacing in the speeches of the leading Nair reformer Mannath Padmanabhan. In the Nair Conference of 1956, he exhorted young Nair men to reap the profits of hard labour, and claimed that only when a man became capable of earning his own income did he qualify to become a householder. He went to the extent of saying, 'at least in our case, a law that prevents the unemployed man—he who lacks the capacity to support his children—from marrying is necessary.' (Pillai 1978: 89). In the well-known presidential address delivered by the renowned communist leader (who entered public life through Malayala brahmin community reformism) E.M.S. Nambutiripad at the Yogakshema Sabha Annual Conference at Ongallur in 1944, young Malayala brahmin men were exhorted to rise up and assume the role of producer and provider of their families (Nambutiripad 1945). Speaking to the Yogakshema Sabha meeting two years later, E.M.S. Nambutiripad urged Malayala brahmins to abandon the old parasitical lifestyle and garner the confidence to support their families through self-earned income and hard labour (Nambutiripad [1946] 1999). This paralleled repeated calls for legal reform that would force men to take responsibility for the economic security and welfare of their wives and children. Early Nair reformers were persistent in this, complaining that brahmin partners (partners in the relatively looser martial tie known as *sambandham*) of Nair women did little to fulfil their duties as fathers and husbands. 'Sahityapanchananan' P.K. Narayana Pillai's speech at the Nair Conference at Kollam in 1922 brought together all the arguments linking the physical and mental condition of women and children, the responsibilities of husbands and the prosperity of the community (Nair 1995: 178–80). The link between full manhood with the capacity to bear full responsibility for the upkeep of one's wife and children was thus cemented not only through legal measures and structural changes that affected the economy and society, but also by innumerable reformist interventions.

Researchers studying the demographic transition in Kerala found some evidence indicating a connection between higher education, lengthening of the waiting period for employment, and age of marriage of men. Writing in the 1970s, T.N. Krishnan remarked that the rise in the age of marriage of women, which seemed to be a major causative factor, might be 'consequent upon a rise in the average age at marriage of males'. He linked this to the improvements in education of men, increased unemployment and the consequent lengthening of the period of waiting for employment (Krishnan 1976: 1223). This was placed in the context of the erosion of traditional support-structures in the wake of extensive socio–economic reforms that altered landownership and family ties, leading to the 'emergence of unitary families in Kerala in place of traditional joint families' (Krishnan 1976: 1223). I have however argued that the assumption of the role of chief provider for one's wife and children by young men here was not just the mechanical effect of certain economic compulsions or the transformation of certain social arrangements. While these are certainly important, it can hardly be forgotten that the ability to maintain a family on one's self-earned income had also become a crucial norm defining adulthood and masculinity itself, such that even those unconstrained by material want increasingly sought to conform with it.

The call to generate and redirect the energies of men into the new family, ascribing to them complete personal and 'natural' responsibility for the upkeep of the family, was decisive in that it enabled the opening up of an agency within the domestic world to which appeals could be made on behalf of the nation. It has been observed that in liberal political thinking, the family is regarded as the natural foundation of civil life and hence of crucial concern for the modern state. However, as it is criss-crossed by other relations—for instance, kin ties, affective connections—it may indeed not be readily and naturally open to the working of the liberal state (Pateman 1989: 21). The father, as head of the family, is thus an important target in the state's efforts to refashion the family—and fatherhood itself—in modern terms. Through him the state would reorder modern domestic space and refashion its inhabitants, and cooperating with this would constitute one of his foremost duties as loyal subject.[3]

In this context, an early manual of the correct upbringing of children, addressed to fathers, written by the modernizing dewan of nineteenth century Travancore, T. Madhava Rao (spelt Madava Row in the text) makes interesting reading (Row 1889). Rao sets about giving 'hints on the training of native children' to fathers, assuming such ready access of fathers to children, that they may easily shape their children's bodies and minds. The appeal to produce healthy and disciplined children is made on behalf of both family and nation (Row 1889: i). Possibly, it assumes sufficient familiarity with modern ideals of individual and collective life amongst father–readers; and this would be one reason why the text was addressed to them in the first place. In late nineteenth century Malayali society, certainly more fathers than mothers, were exposed to such ideas. Very soon, with the spread of modern education and Western values among women in Kerala, such advice would be entirely redirected towards women, and with renewed force. Later, the educated woman was identified as the transforming agent in the family. The early feminists in Malayali society were vociferously pointing out by the late 1920s that it was unfair to exclude women from full citizenship. They advanced their claims on the belief that women deserved full citizenship as they were the appropriate agents for modernizing the family (Devika 2005).

The main body of the text is a detailed account of how to care for the body and mind of the child. This included instructions on proper food, clothing, and hygiene, suggestions regarding the establishment of an economy of rewards and punishments to control the child's actions, the shaping of childrens' minds through words, narratives, and display of emotions. Here the shape to be taken by modern political power is simultaneously etched out with clarity: it is to be the power of fostering life, of which the institution of the modern family is identified as a vital radiating point. In Rao's text, the state is projected as dependent on such non-coercive power, and its thrust is towards transforming the domestic domain in order to adjust it to the new regimen of power; to functionalize it in a different direction. He writes about the limits that may be set to children's play: 'All things that give the child pleasure will do it good. Therefore such pleasurable activities should be curbed only when they cause harm to others. Children must be made to understand that this is the best principle to rule a country, and so our practice must conform to this.' (Row 1889: 4) Interestingly, though this text constantly addresses fathers, it scarcely reminds them of the necessity of providing material support for the family. As the reformers were never tired of reiterating, such access to and authority upon children would be possible only when the father assumed full economic responsibility for their welfare. The altercation between the *karanavar* (the head of the joint family) Panchu Menon and the indigent father of the young boy Shinnan, over his education in O. Chandu Menon's *Indulekha* (1889) is a brilliant literary illustration of this (Menon 1989). This text simply *assumes* that the father's position is already in place, and then proceeds to fine-tune it, and so a reminder of the financial responsibilities of being father/householder does not seem essential. Instead, fathers are instructed in the minute details of childcare. The benevolent father and the benevolent state are projected as exercising the same forms of power. Just as the disciplinary efforts of the benevolent father may be justified as being in the interest of the family, the interventions of the state in society may be justified as precisely in the interest of the nation. He writes: 'The child must be informed time to time that a just government takes care of all the people in the same way as a father cares for his children. The child must know that all people ought to respect the government in the same way children respect their father' (Row 1889: 60). Ultimately, the family is to become into a training ground in which the new form of political power may be encountered in microcosmic form.

These associations gained steady expansion and embellishment in twentieth century Malayali society. Much public discussion on such themes of government, subjecthood, citizenship, social progress, and justice would continue to affirm Rao's vision of the state's moulding of worthy subjects through non-coercive power. Some of this discussion extended his arguments further. A. Gopala Menon's *Samudayolkkarsham* (1924), for instance, dwelt on the duties of the subject of such a state. It recommended that the individual should actively contribute to and cooperate with the efforts of the state to facilitate the self-development of every individual by actualizing their inherent and 'natural' capacities. Individuals were advised to desist from activities that could impede the self-development of others (Menon 1924: 15). Activities that obstructed the state's efforts to guide each one into self-development were deemed to be deserving of punishment. Neglect of the duty of the role of domestic provider figured among these 'socially harmful' faults of the individual. 'Inability to repay debts or provide for the family due to excessive spending or licentious living' is classified among the types of behaviour that affects society as a whole, and not just the individual member or family, (Menon 1924: 17). So also, the shaping of individuals within the family is counted as part of one's 'duty to others':

> Those who have attained maturity and capacity for self-support can gauge their situation, know their desires and fashion their future better that anyone else. Till then, however, many [*others*] will be responsible for [*one's*] self-development. This is how *grihabharanam* [rule of the home]—that is, the protection and culturing of those who are dependent upon oneself—becomes so very important in Man's liberated existence. [Menon 1925: 16.]

Thus in this reckoning, if those entrusted with *grihabharanam* proved to be lax or negligent, the state was completely justified in initiating steps to ensure conformity. In Madhava Rao's terms, such efforts by the state would be fired by the same spirit that infuses a father performing his 'Nature-ordained' duty of correcting his children for their own good. 'Responsible parenthood,' in sum, meant not just the assumption of responsibility for the welfare of one's children, but also one's responsibility to the state.

The modern father and the modern mother bore the burden of 'responsible parenting' equally, but in a uniquely gendered way. Mothers were expected to actively assume the supervision of the bodies, souls, sentiments, and material things within the domestic space. Thus, the science of child-crafting prescribed by Rao soon became projected as an exclusively female concern. New forms of anxieties began to accumulate around mothering as a mode of supervision, evident for instance in the poetry of the prominent poet, Balamani Amma.[4] The chief means of actualizing the mother/homemaker prescribed was education, which was expected to both generate fresh energy within women and to channel it back into the home. From being *pettamma* (mother-as-bearer), the mother is now raised to being the major agent of reproduction. It was the Protestant missionaries first, and then enthusiastic local reformers' who took up this cause with considerable zest and vigour. In this light, earlier expressions of motherly love and devotion appeared passive and pointless. An author remarked on the difference as follows:

> Due to their ignorance, our mothers have no idea about their place and responsibility. Though many Hindus, through false fasts, and Christians and Muslims, through vows and donations, seek to attain motherhood, they have no idea of the sacrifice and austerity necessary for the attainment of true motherhood.... If one desires to be a mother, severe austerities are to be practiced. Only then will the sleeping Indian nation arise into wakefulness ... [Amma 1925: 3.]

A wide gulf appears to separate the two forms of mothering, earlier ones being relegated to superficial show. The essence of motherliness is now identified to lie in the modern mother's desire to shape her children into disciplined and rational Individuals. Indeed, 'liberating' children from the 'earlier animal-like maternal love', to some early advocates of birth control, seemed no less than a precondition for fashioning them as individuals, and birth control appeared to be the appropriate tool:

> Careful observers are quite sure to opine that the love for children has only increased after the acceptance of birth control. It may be possible to admit that the earlier animal-like motherly affection expressed in kisses and cuddles, with little concern for cleanliness, nutrition etc., has decreased with birth control. Today's mother who has limited the number of her children is striving very hard to provide them with favourable circumstances as far as possible. [[Author not mentioned] 'Santananiyantranam' [Birth Control], *The Mahila* 1932: 373.]

Indeed, from the early twentieth century onwards, a huge volume of writing sought to cleanse local women of their 'passive' motherliness, point out the defects in their mental equipment, and suggest better ways of inculcating discipline among the young. Many women reformers, like the redoubtable K. Chinnamma, devoted considerable energies to this (see, for instance, Chinnamma [1913] 2005: 29–36). This effort was made in the interest of both the family and other groups such as the community or the nation. In the article quoted above, a new standard of judging the strength of character came to the fore: a willingness to sacrifice oneself for the nation. Rejecting the argument that single children tended to be weak and selfish, the above-quoted author wrote: 'The accusation that such infants may become weak is refuted by the fact that many thousands of only children joined the army during the last war for the defense of the land.' (*Mahila* 1932: 373). The nation thus enters the mother–child intimacy. The mother's loving attention must not simply generate pleasure-for-itself; it must be strictly yoked to the production of useful subjects for the nation.

The new domestic ideology and the new notions of maternal responsibility spread in the early decades of the twentieth century through the widening network of schools, which registered a remarkable increase in girl pupils in these times (Jeffrey 2003). However, equally—or perhaps more important were the informal networks—a fact less noticed in conventional accounts of Kerala's educational history. Non-formal education through institutions such as the Mahila Samajams (women's associations) which often worked very closely with reformist organizations, schools, churches, was indeed saturated with the new domestic ideology. (Devika 1999: 86–90).

These were institutions destined to be promoted by the modernizing state, especially after Indian independence. They were to function as an important area in which birth limitation was smoothly blended into, made part of, the role of the supervising, efficient modern mother. In the community development project of the 1950s, women were largely addressed primarily as caregivers for the family, and much effort was directed to improving such skills, adding some encouragement to income generation through home-based economic activities. The central social welfare boards established social welfare extension projects and encouraged the setting up of Mahila Samajams in the Second Plan, generally focused on domestic concerns (Eapen 2000: 4). In 1966, about 2000 Mahila Samajams existed in the state (GoK 1966: 345). In any case, by these times, the state was convinced of the widespread familiarity of women with the new child rearing practices. The authors of the Fourth Five Year-Plan (1969–74) for Kerala commented as follows when discussing the proposed Family and Child Welfare Centres:

> One of the basic assumptions of the project is that the majority of rural mothers do not have any formal education and that they should be educated effectively by carrying [out] necessary training in home craft and mother craft. This position is not wholly applicable to Kerala. The rural mothers of this part of the country have sufficient understanding of the art of bringing up their children and the emphasis on mother craft may not be relevant. [State Planning Board, Go K 1969: 248.]

Thus, the propaganda of the FPP had very well prepared soil in which to root itself, as by the 1960s, the ideal of 'responsible parenting' had gained widespread circulation in Malayali society, especially among women with a minimum education. It was presented as an effective means of shaping individuals by making possible the concentration of the material and mental resources of the parents upon fewer children. FP, by the late 1950s, had gained a place within the social 'uplift' efforts of the government that sought to equip women to be better homemakers. The women's camps conducted as part of the community development programme at the Block level in the late 1950s, it is pointed out, intended to introduce women to such subjects as 'care of the family, health, nutrition, cooking, childcare, family planning, poultry farming, kitchen gardening … ' (Nanu 1960: 188–9). At the same time, propagating FP was projected as an ideal way of serving the nation. In 1966, a Mahila Samajam of Kuttali panchayat reportedly set apart one day in a month for the 'service of the nation' in the same spirit in which devotional vows/fasts—*vratams*—are offered. This day was to be devoted to 'offering voluntary labour in construction activities, taking part in family planning work, planting kitchen gardens and so on' (*Malayala Manorama* 6 April 1969: 3). However, FP was certainly not portrayed as an exclusively womanly preoccupation, also being depicted, in innumerable instances, as the major tool for the fulfilment of the duty of the father/householder to support his wife and children upon his self-earned income.

While the commonality of interest between the family and the nation was continually stressed, it was sometimes suggested that mentioning the nation's interest only after the gains to the family through FP was strategically wise. That is, some FP publicists found it unwise to project the acceptance of FP as a service to the nation, and that 'even those who have no great interest in the welfare of the Nation will have concern about their own children' (Babu 1960: I). The bureaucratic-technocratic accusation that 'improvident maternity' represented anti-social and anti-national behaviour stressed that the nation was nothing other than a 'large family', the interests of which ought to predominate over those of the individual family (for instance, public statements by R.A. Gopalaswamy, cited in Petersen 1966). The alleged commonality of interests between these institutions was rarely critically scrutinized. Even the Catholic Church in the 1960s and '70s warmly endorsed 'responsible parenting', 'responsible parenthood', and birth limitation albeit without 'artificial' birth control, (see, Manikkatan 1972).

To reject it could even be interpreted as outright selfishness. Thus an appeal issued in 1966 from the 'outside' to the 'inside', by 'prominent citizens' to 'all married couples in Kerala' pointed out that the importance of FP lay precisely in that it was not merely a measure to assure financial stability but a 'national need' (*Matrubhumi* 5 September 1966: 6). For the state, however, projecting FP as primarily benefiting the individual family held some very solid advantage. To project it as sacrifice on the part of the individual in the interest of the nation would leave some space for the individual to make a claim for special consideration from the state. This was clearly evident in the aftermath of the highly successful mass vasectomy camp held at Ernakulam in 1971, which was widely portrayed as a *Yagna:* 'a sacred, concerted and concentrated effort involving the sacrifice of the participants and the public at the altar of the future welfare of the nation' (Kumar 1971: 29). Given this orientation, some of the developments that followed the mass vasectomy camp at Ernakulam in 1971 seem particularly interesting. Accompanying news reports that around 1500 persons who had undergone vasectomy at the camp were hospitalized with infections and bleeding, there was a report that efforts were on to organize a 'union' of the *vandheekrtar*, i.e. the sterilized (*Matrubhumi* 12 August 1971: 5). A meeting held by the *vandheekrtar* of Kanjoor and adjoining areas presided over by a certain T.K. Prabhakaran apparently decided to form an organization called Kerala Vandheekrta Union (*Matrubhumi* 12 August 1971: 5). The statement issued by M.R. Nanappan, convenor of the Working Committee elected in the meeting reportedly said:

> The sterilized people are those who have voluntarily committed themselves to the cause of preventing the excessive increase in population facing India, and if they are not to be ignored then such an organisation is necessary … many who underwent sterilization surgery are mentally and physically upset today. Many of them, who were capable of hard labour, now struggle

to work ... We must find solutions to all this. [*Matrubhumi* 12 August 1971: 5.]

Such claims upon the state, made on the basis of sacrifices rendered, could easily become invalid once it was affirmed that FP was fundamentally the need of the individual family, pegged to individual happiness, specified as the ability to fulfill one's 'natural' obligations as father/householder or mother/homemaker. Besides happiness, the need for FP was also pegged to one's sense of honour and decency. The well-known FP propagandist, A.P. Udayabhanu, persistently argued that the success of FP propaganda lay in linking 'shame' and 'lack of responsibility' to large families and elevating the acceptance of birth limitation into a cultural norm. He wrote, 'To parade around pregnancy beyond the third child, one suspects, is already being looked down in society. The time in which such persons will be derided as shameless and irresponsible is not distant.' (Udayabhanu 1967: 4.)

The alliance between the individual family and the nation projected in the FP propaganda dissolved the interests of communities into the background. Indeed, the community movements, which were a formidable presence in Malayali society and completely committed to the politics of numbers, did not really obstruct the acceptance of family limitation. It was not as if suspicion and concern about the effects of the widespread acceptance of FP on community politics were never voiced. Nevertheless, it was the community movements that had forcefully propagated the ideal of 'responsible parenting' in Malayali society since the early twentieth century. Their own vision of the ideal modern community of the future was inevitably one in which the individual family supported by the labour of the parents figured as the keystone. In the 1960s, prominent community movements were lending support to family planning activities. The prominent Nair leader Mannath Padmanabhan was making speeches that actively advocated 'responsible parenting' through birth limitation.[5] The Mahila Samajams and other fora of the Nair Service Society and the Sree Narayana Dharma Paripalana Yogam were also aiding FP work (Peetambaran 1969: 209–10). The Catholic

Church, notwithstanding its uncompromising rejection of 'artificial' birth control, did approve of family limitation through other means, and that too in the interest of both the family and the nation (Manikkathan 1972). The signatories of the appeal for FP by 'prominent citizens' in 1966 were all from diverse communities and faiths, apparently uniting in the interest of the home and the nation. They included luminaries such as K.P.S. Menon, prominent Muslim leaders T.A. Abdulla and P.K. Kunhu, the Nair reformer Mannath Padmanabhan, the Congressman C.M. Stephen, the communist leader T.V. Thomas, the veteran Congresswoman A.V. Kuttimalu Amma, and others (*Matrubhumi* 5 September 1966: 6).

Thus, by highlighting the shaping of children into fully-fledged individuals as the right way of raising children, 'responsible parenting' significantly increased the quantum of energy required to raise a child, and demanded it as a 'natural', gendered obligation from parents. This, in itself, was a condition directing parents towards family limitation. At the same time, in and through 'responsible parenting', the modern family was imagined as fully amenable to control and direction by the modern state. Early enough, the widespread acceptance of 'responsible parenting' was recognized as being crucial to the actualization of the developed nation of the future, and citizens were directed towards assuming it as their duty towards the nation. Through 'responsible parenting', it became possible to project the emergent political rationality of the new state as being quite distanced from politics itself, as a magnified altruism. The family was to remain open to correction by the state whenever it seemed to fail in the adequate performance of the task of child-crafting assigned to it, precisely because the state was projected as occupying the position of the benevolent father vis-à-vis society. By the mid-twentieth century, such ideas had gained quite remarkable circulation, especially among the newly educated, in Malayali society. The publicists of the FPP of the 1960s would abundantly draw upon them. In turn, they would increase the velocity of the circulation of these ideas as well as take them to groups placed further away from the modern educated classes.[6]

Building the Individual's Castle

Notwithstanding the higher costs of child-raising implied in 'responsible parenting', it is still quite difficult to pinpoint this as the crucial condition that made FP acceptable to very diversely placed social groups in mid-twentieth century Malayali society. As seen earlier, for instance in George Mathen's words cited above, 'responsible parenting' was clearly associated with the large family and not the small one. What are then the conditions that predisposed agents to link 'responsible parenting' with the small family? Concomitant with the rise of 'responsible parenting' was the notion of family subsistence, as involving the achievement of a balance between scarce means and ceaseless wants. The crystallization of such a notion, along with 'responsible parenting', as a common sense view among groups of people could have been significant in their gradual internalization of the modern family as the small family. However, given that the 'initial conditions' for each social caste-/class-group in Kerala were distinct, we may suppose that there were many, and not necessarily connected, routes by which such associations as the above were built. Thus, if this understanding of family subsistence solidified in certain groups through their desire towards salaried employment, others may have encountered it under very different circumstances. For instance, the insecurities about the future that began to appear on the horizon of existence of the agricultural workers in the 1970s could well have served as another such path. This also does not suggest that the understanding of 'means' or 'ends' was unitary across social groups. Much more work will need to be done before we understand these distinct paths. This section attempts to tentatively open this inquiry.

One may start, perhaps, with the question how the new élite of twentieth century Kerala—principally from the three dominant communities, the Nair, the Ezhava, and the Syrian Christians—arrived at this new conception of family survival. It is now argued quite strongly that the fertility decline in Kerala may not have been the result of greater female autonomy, even though high levels of schooling does have a marked impact (Rajan et al. 1996). Here I take a cue from demographers who suggest that female schooling (and consequently, female age at marriage) is associated with male schooling and employment (Bhat and Rajan 1990; Rajan et al. 1996), to focus on both women and femininity, and men and masculinity, in discussing the shaping of the small family norm. Thus, it may be relevant here to make a brief foray into the history of dominant masculinities in Kerala, for these new ideals were deeply entangled with the emergent ideals of family and its upkeep. Examining late nineteenth and early twentieth century writings, one may notice that the question of masculinity is raised prominently in relation to both the public and domestic domains. The new ideals of masculine subjectivity that were being advanced often carried within the ideal citizen–subject. In the contexts of community reformism and national progress, men were often exhorted to realize their 'manhood' by becoming able producers of wealth and useful subjects of the nation (Devika 1999: 93–5). Nevertheless, the ideal new man was not exclusively imagined within the space of the nation-state. The joint family often provided the space against which the new man was defined, especially in many late nineteenth century novels (Nair [1890] 1988; Menon [1889] 1989). In both ways of constructing the ideal man, however, the capacity to remain free from dependence on traditional support structures, including feudal patronage and the joint family, was equally emphasized. Thus the ideal man was defined as someone capable of opposing entrenched powers. These ideas continued to be developed in the early twentieth century. A discussion of ideal masculinity published in 1933 waxed as follows about the 'real' man: 'Today [we] need a man who is capable of maintaining his individuality in the midst of the group, who has not the slightest hesitation to say 'no' when the whole world says 'yes'. All fields, including those of industry, trade and art seek such a man.' (Menon and Menon 1933: 1.)

Of these, the first was clearly implicated in the larger collectivity, especially the nation-state and the community. In Malayali society, reflections on how the individual ought to be ideally implicated within larger social collectivities (community, church, nation) appeared almost alongside the earliest articulations of 'responsible parenting' in the late nineteenth and early twentieth centuries.

The modern collectivity seemed to call for *subjects* who participate in reshaping the collectivity, and not merely those born into it by chance. As the abundance of material wealth was seen to be an important criterion marking the ideal worldly modern collectivity, this active role was often understood as involving the energetic pursuit of material wealth, or at least, achieving material self-sufficiency. Members were constantly urged to contribute 'positively' by becoming industrious and efficient producers. Sufficiently early in colonial rule, this worked as a standard for assessing the worth of social groups. Groups who appeared to deviate drastically from this ideal were noticed and commented upon. Francis Buchanan, commenting on the Nayadis of Malabar, used precisely this standard, and voiced exactly this concern. Calling them parasites on the land, a 'wretched tribe ... buffeted and abused by everyone', he swore on 'both compassion and justice', that they should be 'compelled to gain a livelihood by honest industry, and thus 'elevated somewhat more nearly to the rank of men' (Buchanan [1807] 1988: 144).[7] However, even groups that were self-sufficient—for instance, peasants—could be reckoned as non-productive from the nation-state's perspective if they failed to produce a surplus. The First Prince of Travancore, in a speech delivered in 1874, quoted at length from an Administrative Report of Travancore that presented a glowing picture of self-sufficiency and contentment reigning in the 'rural Arcadia of Travancore', only to argue that '... the very contentment and conservation have proved the greatest obstacle to industrial progress ... It has seldom or never entered the thoughts of the peasant or those better than him, to endeavour to make two blades of grass grow where only one does now' (Varma 1874: 3–4). Clearly, this was hardly a recommendation for further frugality on the part of the peasant or the aspiring citizen–subject. It was even being argued that a change to a more consumption-oriented lifestyle would actually boost production of surplus through the creation of new needs. V. Nagam Aiya, well-known bureaucrat and the author of the *Travancore Manual*, struck this vein when he complained about agriculture in Travancore: 'What we know and have known for a long time is a condition of perennial want in greater or lesser degree ... the lazy and miserable Travancore *ryot* ekes out a miserable existence, and his inexpensive clothing, food and drink contribute their quota to his general inefficiency …' (Aiya 1909: 3–4).

Nagam Aiya's exasperated admission was that he would have tolerated an expensive lifestyle if it shook the *ryot* out of his relaxed attitude and ushered in market-oriented production to solve both 'perennial want' and the needs of the nation. This plaint was of long duration. Writing close to mid-century, T.K. Krishna Menon voiced the same complaint for Cochin (Menon 1948). The same solution figured in the proposals of development-initiators. Spencer Hatch, the director of Rural Demonstration and Training in Travancore in the 1930s, which aimed at rationalizing village life, prescribed this in 1932. His method was to encourage the modernization of agriculture and allied activities, and the cooperative system in production and marketing. The money economy and the social circumstance in which one would need 'more income with which to purchase the necessities of life' (Hatch 1932: 99) was assumed to be well in place. The integration of the rural poor into the market-based economy is the solution to their poverty, and the formation of a larger collectivity, what he calls the community, is the principal means to this end (Hatch 1932: 11). At the same time, all these schemes for local improvement must be 'a real factor in the welfare of the society of which the group is a part—community, state or nation.' (Hatch 1932: 125). Of course, these arguments for capitalism are quite familiar: the flourishing of modern collectivities—especially the nation-state—was viewed as pivoted upon increasing production and consumption, expected to intensify each other. The subjects of the nation-state were required to actively foster both.

The second, however, was implicated much more in the modern family. It is perhaps pertinent to remember that the construction of the modern man in early Malayalam novels is framed by their textual staging of the confrontation between the entrenched order and the emergent modern one. The ideal man, thus, is depicted to be in confrontation with the established order, and armed with the material authority of the colonial/ state power, and the intellectual authority of Western knowledge. He is, most often, employed in colonial institutions of rule or learning, and thus needs little support from traditional institutions to survive. The struggle leads to the constitution of the modern home into which entrenched forces may only minimally encroach. This household is supported by the father/householder's income, derived from mostly non-traditional sources, often from service in colonial institutions.

In one of the early Malayalam novels, these two modern ideals of masculinity come into direct conflict, and the issue of choosing the better one is dealt with. This is *Parangodiparinayam,* which openly lampoons the hankering after modern professions by modern-educated Malayali men. It represents ideal man as a skilled producer of material wealth who is also able to make thoroughly rational judgements on the utility of the different kinds of importation from the West (Menon [1892] 1985). This, however did not mean that the father/householder was banished into oblivion; quite the contrary. Indeed, the ideal male figure, Pangasha Menon, is *both* an efficient producer and a capable householder. The point is that the ideal of father/householder is never eclipsed in the contest between the efficient wealth-producer and the educated professional in defining ideal modern manhood. The ability to build a space relatively insulated from the entrenched powers seemed fundamental; the major differences centred on the most effective means of realizing this. In those times and in those texts, employment in the emergent political, cultural, and economic institutions was identified as both liberating, and enabling the realization of a certain 'manliness'.

The desire for modern education and salaried employment was to become an abiding feature of Malayali modernity, especially among social groups and families with some access to material resources. Examining public discourse in Kerala in the early twentieth century right up to the present, one may see that this is a theme that was most discussed. Even in communities in which thrift and labour were emphasized early, clear shifts seem to have occurred over the course of the twentieth century. Remarking on the patterns of upwardly mobile behaviour among the Ezhavas, Fillipo and Caroline Osella remark that now the former ideals are at odds with new 'mobility ambitions demanding high spending on children, disdain for labour and the pursuit of pleasure' (Osella and Osella 2000: 248). They link this with the dominant masculine, which they identify in the householder: 'over the twentieth century, the cultural figure of the Hindu householder has become merged with the bourgeois pater familias and revitalised as the consuming man of substance.' (Osella and Osella 2000: 245). Such changes have been subsumed 'within this century's totalizing time-narrative of 'progress', and they observe that 'increasingly in Kerala as a whole, the referent for the young men is the world of paid employment'. (Osella and Osella 2000: 245).

The Osellas are referring to the 1990s, but from about the 1920s, one begins to encounter sharp criticisms of the increasing demand for salaried employment among the newly educated classes. This was found to be alienating people from both manual labour as well as self-employment. Writing in 1934, the noted humourist E.V. Krishna Pillai wrote about that new item of clothing, the shirt, which was the very symbol of the new educated classes: 'The shirt has certain disadvantages. He cannot bear the sight of the pickaxe or the shovel. Fields, crops, garden land—these are his inveterate enemies. He cannot bear the sight of paddy. Tapioca, yams, millets—all these are alien to him.' (Pillai [1934] 1987: 187.) The Unemployment Enquiry Committee of Travancore of 1928 noted a strong reluctance among the educated to undertake physical labour (*Report of the Unemployment Enquiry Committee* 1928: 28). In 1940, N.J. Nair issued 'A Plea for a New Outlook in Travancore', in which he decried the widespread tendency of educated young people to swarm around government jobs and recommended that the dignity of manual labour be raised by transforming it through science and technology (Nair 1940: 57). Indeed, the persistence of the arguments against the attraction for salaried employment over the decades is remarkable indeed. Past the mid-twentieth century, the attraction for salaried employment continued to be strongly felt and frequently commented upon in public fora. The reluctance to undertake independent initiatives in productive activities and the attraction for employment was characterized as an unfortunate feature of modernity, and different causes identified for it: traditional conservatism, laziness, bureaucratic indifference, or labour militancy. (Strangely, however, the shallowness of the critique of caste in Malayali society is never mentioned.) Newspapers wavered between demanding that the government satisfy the desire of the educated for employment, and exhorting the educated to give up their sterile desire for employment, and take to the virile desire for productive efficiency. *Matrubhumi* in 1970 lamented as follows on the inability of Malayali engineers to undertake fresh industrial ventures on their own:

> Another solution is that engineers should start some industries. The government is willing to support all such efforts.... But it is said that not enough engineers have come forward to take advantage of opportunities and concessions. One can only say that this is the curse of this land. Everyone wants jobs in the government or in some company. No one is ready to start something new or engage in productive enterprise. The guts and confidence for such initiative is lacking. [*Matrubhumi* 5 March 1970: 4.]

In short, the dominant masculine ideal that seemed most appealing to large sections of the new élite was that of the householder who supported his family through self-earned income through employment. The reason why it has gained such overwhelming presence in Kerala has not yet been explored in much detail. However, the breakdown of joint families, the severe economic insecurities of the Great Depression and the Second World War period, and the lack of substantial economic growth post-Independence may be of crucial importance when we attempt to explain this.[8] Also of great importance is the failure of most political movements in Kerala to overcome the hierarchy implicit in effective mental/manual division of work, and thus mental work came to exclusively signify gentility. I want to argue that the crystallization of dominant masculinity in these terms crucially helped the entrenchment of the new notion of family subsistence among the new Malayali élites.

It must also be noted that such ideals were beginning to circulate very rapidly between different social strata, aided by the expanding literacy and popular media like the cinema. Modern education, and on its heels, employment, continued to appear to be the panacea for poverty and inequality, and the eventual source of social and economic security, for an ever-greater number of social groups, especially those in the lowest rungs of the entrenched social hierarchy, and even among the newly-found organizations of the labouring classes. A pamphlet published by the Chirakkal Taluk peasant union in 1938 raised the issue of the indebtedness and pauperization of the agricultural labourers. However, 'their ultimate sorrow lay in the fact that, 'Though we struggle/ Are we able to dress our children even in rags/ And put a slate and pencil in their hands' (quoted in Menon 1994: 144). Much later, researchers have found precisely the same aspirations among the poor in Kerala, of providing their children with some education and a steady job with regular income (and not higher but intermittent wages) (Saradamoni 1992: 167). Going by the numerous accounts from the autobiographies of individuals who lived through these times, salaried employment, especially in the government, seemed to be the sure guarantee of upward social mobility (for instance, see Amma 1968: 66). Women too seemed to be no different in seeking salaried employment, and identifying it as the chief aim and goal of modern education, as the Statham Committee on educational reforms in Travancore (1933) noted. The root cause of this tendency was identified in the propensity to see education not as something of intrinsic cultural value alone but as 'a direct means of securing employment and competing with men in the open market'. (*Report of the Travancore Educational Reforms Committee* 1933: 256–66). For women too, modern education and salaried employment were sometimes identified as the most reliable means of at least partial deliverance from oppressive patriarchal social arrangements, as, for instance, in the writings of radicals like K. Saraswati Amma (Devika 2002) and Kuttippuzha Krishna Pillai (Pillai [1941, 1944] 1990), in the 1940s and '50s. Nevertheless, this was not to proliferate; instead, women's paid work outside the home was gradually reconciled with women's domestic responsibilities. If salaried employment frequently appeared to be the most feasible way of realizing modern manhood, efforts were on, early enough in the twentieth century, to argue that it was not necessarily inimical to modern womanhood, and to the role of the modern mother/homemaker (though not made central to it, as in the case of modern manhood) (Devika 2006). By the 1960s, the necessity of an active economic contribution to the household income by the mother came to be increasingly endorsed as a necessity for the maintenance of the self-supporting nuclear family. This formed yet another argument in favour of family limitation, stressing the opportunity costs of time and energy spent on childbearing and rearing for the woman and her family.

Besides, newspapers of these decades report several instances that reveal deep anxieties and insecurity among the young and the educated about the difficulty of finding employment. These generally point at a socio–economic milieu in which traditional social-support mechanisms were steadily dwindling, initiative to generate employment seemed lacking, and the necessity of finding one's own income was being projected as crucial for both family survival (for women) and the attainment of (male) adulthood. *Matrubhumi*'s report of an interview conducted at Kollam for the recruitment of five policewomen, for which 2000 applications were received, is particularly telling. Some of the 385 candidates selected for the interview told *Matrubhumi*'s reporter that it was sheer material need and lack of other options that had prompted them to apply for work in the police (*Matrubhumi* 21 February 1968: 4).

The FP propaganda seized particularly on the anxieties that were bred by the conception of the modern family as a consumption-oriented unit supported by a wage/salary, primarily of the father/householder. Here we may draw upon the insights of demographers who remark about the relation between income and fertility, that the demand for children may rise with income, 'at least until changing tastes, changing aspirations and new ideas about quantity–quality trade-offs reduce these effects.' (Jeffrey and Basu 1996: 36). Jeffrey and Basu observe that one could well assume that 'declines in child mortality might make mothers more confident about their child-raising abilities, and more willing to bring up an additional child, at least until other cost increasing factors step in' (Basu 1996: 37). As remarked earlier, change in favour of fewer children and rising costs of child-raising has been observed for Kerala (for instance, Mahadevan and Sumangala 1987: 41; 64–5; 72); here we draw out the implications of the changes observed. Representations of the ideal (new élite) family in the 1960s centred upon high consumption.[9] One instance is particularly interesting: an essay that won the first prize in a contest for women conducted by *Malayala Manorama* on the topic 'The Family I Dream Of' (*Malayala Manorama* 27 November 1970: 6). In the detailed description of the ideal family, it is the concrete space inhabited by the family—the rooms of the house—and then the objects found essential that are foregrounded. Among these are counted the radio, the fan, electric iron, the meat safe, the pressure cooker, and the dressing table, which are cited to be 'no longer articles of ostentation' but necessities. Following this is an assessment of the family size within which it would be possible to maintain such a lifestyle. As may be expected, FP is warmly endorsed. This order of priority in describing the ideal family was certainly not limited to this single text. The condemnation of those who favoured artificial contraception as consumerists steeped in worldly pleasures, heard since the 1930s onwards,[10] seems to have simply burnt itself out. What had once appeared to be mindless luxury came to be acknowledged as a necessity for decent existence, and birth limitation looked less like a path to overindulgence and more like the royal road to the genteel life. Indeed, it has been observed that the small family almost inevitably formed part of the representations of high-consumption oriented 'good life' in the West. Writing about pictorial advertisements in the US during the 1920s and '30s, Roland Marchand notes that a picture of a larger family was extremely rare, probably because it might indicate the lack of middle-class status (Marchand 1985: 164–205).

In such a family as described in the prize-winning article mentioned above, the benefits of FP are patently self-evident. 'Responsible parenting' was, in any case, an intrinsic part of new élite ambitions for upward mobility. The limits of consumption that a fixed salary set, and the rising consumption aspirations ensured that it was all the more possible to talk of family subsistence as revolving around relatively limited means and steadily multiplying wants, and of children as economic liabilities. When 'responsible parenting' was conducted within the consumption-oriented household supported by a limited, if regular, salary, the wisdom of family limitation could hardly be missed. Many acceptors during the mass sterilization campaign of the early 1970s cited this as their reason for acceptance. *Matrubhumi* quoted an industrial worker welcoming FP in 1970:

> My parents had nine children including myself. My father was a teacher. Due to the economic difficulties in my family, I had to give up studies at the age of seventeen and join the army. It was not ill health or incompetence at studies that hindered my education. It was sheer economic want that placed hurdles before me ... At least my children must be spared of this misfortune. [*Matrubhumi* 27 June 1970: 2]

These were also times in which the poor were also being increasingly drawn into the discourse of family limitation. Traditional obligations binding different groups had either collapsed, or were in the process of collapsing, with the result that food and shelter seems to have become increasingly insecure. Much earlier, birth limitation had been suggested by relief workers trying to alleviate the dire situation in the wake of near-famine conditions in the early 1940s, during the Second World War (Jeffrey 2003: 196). The traces of the insecurities engendered by the erosion of the traditional social and economic arrangements are not difficult to find. In 1968, *Kerala Kaumudi* reported R.S. Unny speaking in the Kerala State Legislative Assembly about the difficulties in securing housing faced by landless tenants in the aftermath of the ban on eviction since 1957. Demanding a housing scheme for them, he pointed out that

> Though eviction has been banned and *kutikidappukar* [tenants] have been protected since 1957, the situation today is that more people cannot become *kutikidappukar*. The result is that more than one family resides in the same

> *kuti* [hut]. If there is a god, then that god alone knows how difficult it is for such people to fulfill primary human needs thus squeezed into a single *kuti*. [*Kerala Kaumudi* 9 November 1968: 5.]

Other accounts, such as those of the well-known journalist and author of the 1960s, Pavanan, illuminate the desperate struggle for survival among groups increasingly cut off from land and traditional survival strategies. His pen-portraits of 'ordinary Malayalis' of the 1960s, evoke images of extreme poverty and suffering among the poor, trying to fend for themselves in a situation in which work was neither easy to find, nor sufficiently remunerative to support even minimum needs (Pavanan 1967). The intense conflicts over redistribution in the agrarian sector continued well past the land reforms, and these were clearly tied to the grim question of survival in an agrarian society in which a sizeable class of agricultural labourers, over a third of the entire rural workforce in Kerala in 1971, depended on a landholding class, eighty-five per cent of which owned under an acre of land (Heller 1999; Tharamangalam 1981; Kannan 1988; Isaac 1982).

At the same time, the ideas of the importance of the family and the primary responsibility of the husband towards providing economic support to his family were beginning to achieve greater circulation among the poorest and most deprived. To mention just one such area: we find these firmly institutionalized, for instance, in the *Report of the Minimum Wages Committee for Cashew Industry* of 1953, commissioned by the government of Travancore-Cochin (cited in Lindberg 2001). It justified the nuclear family as supportive of a disciplined and thrift-oriented life, with the husband a responsible provider. Proclaiming such a family in which the husband provided for the wife and children to be desirable, it legitimized the discrepancy between the wages of male and female workers, holding that women were not expected to maintain their husbands (Lindberg 2001). On the other hand, increasingly, women who worked for wages were being represented as primarily mothers engaged in paid work to enhance the family's income. Some research on the desires, aspirations and ideals of lower-class families supported by unskilled labour, reveals that the father/

householder-mother/homemaker axis seems to have crystallized among these couples, at least in the realm of ideals (University of Kerala 1965: 43–44). In other words, it became gradually possible to articulate the ideology of 'responsible parenting' in the context of the poor working class family. Thus, the FPP's arrival could not have been better timed. On the one hand, questions of everyday survival seemed to be pressing the poorest sections hard; on the other hand, 'responsible parenting' was rising in the horizon of working class life, issuing forth from a whole range of sites ranging from governmental institutions to trade union struggles to popular theatre and cinema. Parvati Ayappan, who was actively involved in promoting FP in the late 1960s and '70s, candidly advances this:

> These are times in which ordinary people are being tormented by heavy burdens of responsibility and the severity of economic difficulties. Everyone desires to be liberated from this situation. Everyone is now convinced that adopting the policy of family limitation is the easy way towards this.... Plentiful gifts ... Each person gets around a hundred rupees as money, things, and ration rice. This is indeed a great boon in these months of *Mithunam–Karkadakam* [June–July] which are the months of difficulty.... [Ayappan 1971: 5.]

In its editorials, *Kerala Kaumudi* reminded its readers that family limitation was no longer a strategy of the rich to preserve their wealth, but the single most important solution to the problem of the survival of the poor. Pointing to the extreme insecurity that seemed to have pervaded Malayali society, it claimed:

> If Kerala, which has been generously endowed by Nature is to overcome today's calamities and once again become the ancient *Mavelinadu* [the realm of the legendary Malayali king Maveli, in which people are said to have enjoyed total security of life], population increase must be consciously curbed. There is not enough rice gruel to give surviving children, no cloth to wear, no roof to sleep under, no means to educate—if parents produce more children fully aware of this state of affairs, then they are committing a heinous crime. [5 August 1967: 2.]

There is some reason to believe that the waning of communal

forms of life-sustenance (however meagre), and dependence on wage-income may have been the key conditions that underlay the gradual acceptance of FP among the agricultural proletariat. This waning may have taken place quite gradually. For instance, Patrick Heller has argued that the Kerala Agricultural Workers Act was really a granting of 'legal sanction to customary right'. It gave legal status of 'permanent worker', with a guaranteed right to employment, to any labourer who had worked in a particular landowner's property, by custom, contract, or otherwise (Heller 1999: 138–9). He also mentions that for the successful cultivators, this was little more than an extension of the older patron–client relation (Heller 1999: 143). It is the gradual attrition of permanency, apparently 'traded for wage increases', that he actually records (Heller 1999: 145). It cannot be glibly assumed that the land reforms ended traditional forms of patronage and set in place the economic emancipation of the poor (see, for instance, Schenk-Sandbergen 1988; Nieuwenhuys 1991). Though often treated by non-academic admirers of the Kerala Model as an aside, economists have cautioned sufficiently early about placing too much importance on education and health in fertility reduction. They pointed to the possibility that the decline in the fertility of the poor may have been an effect of the 'deepening of the distress among the poor'. They reminded that there was indirect evidence for this: 'An examination of the occupational distribution of sterilized persons shows that nearly 60 per cent of the males and nearly 38 per cent of the females belonged to the groups of unskilled workers and agricultural labourers during the period 1965 to 1974. Moreover, their proportion in the total number of sterilizations appears to have increased during the period 1966–74 over that during 1955–65'. (Panikar et al. 1978: 68–9). Other work too indicates the possibility that FP acceptance by the poor could have been a strategy for survival (for instance, Gulati 1981: 49, 74–5; van der Werff 1992: 125). It has been pointed out that the expected gain in agricultural growth through land reforms did not really fructify (Panikar et al. 1978: 55), and that the erstwhile tenants found other profitable use for the land they gained, and that status–mobility was not entirely free of new concerns, especially about the future of children: 'Agricultural labourers were forced to think of other means of survival for their children. They sent their children to school and tried thus to acquire jobs in the organized sector. Their ability to do so was limited in spite of government-guaranteed reservations.' (Tharakan 2002: 359) The snowballing of these new anxieties of survival, focused around the home, into the 1980s and '90s, has been documented (den Uyl 1995; Morrison 1997: 61–87; Ramanathaiyer and Macpherson 2000).

Besides, consumption-oriented lifestyles were also reaching the economically weaker sections of the people. By the 1960s, these were gradually becoming the standard by which village life was assessed, and condemned. We have little information on exactly how these new desires spread into an increasing number of groups, but certain traces remain in writings. One such is to be found in Pavanan's pen-portraits of 'ordinary Malayalis' of the 1960s, which focused on agricultural labourers, plantation workers, cashew workers, and others. In this he records the changes in lifestyle in a small farmer's household in rural Kerala and remarks:

> For sure, in the interior of Tamil Nadu, Gujarat or Uttar Pradesh, an agricultural family of the economic standards of Kunhiraman Nair's household will not have needs of this sort. However, for the great majority of agricultural families in Kerala not all this can be dismissed as unnecessary expenditure. Using scented soap, collyrium, silk clothes, going to the movies, using talcum powder, all have become common even among farming families. [Pavanan 1967: 59–60.]

The FPP amply cashed in on this, taking this vision of the genteel life to the poorer classes. The gifts given away at FP camps in the early 1970s were almost symbolic of the higher-consumption lifestyle that a smaller family seemed to promise: stainless steel vessels, cooking stoves, watches, suitcases, radios, clocks, bicycles, electric torches and fans, lamps, and the like (Kumar 1971: 40). FP publicists stressed the necessity of family limitation in spurring even further the consumption-oriented lifestyle attained by the better-off: 'Today, the living standards of our middle class has gone up considerably in comparison with earlier times. Most of them want to see it go further up. There is no other reason why they display greater interest in Family Planning than any other group.' (Ayappan 1971: 5).

'Responsible parenting,' which demanded much greater energy, time, and wealth for child rearing; the solidifying of the recognition of family subsistence as involving limited means and steadily expanding wants among the new élite through new ideals of masculinity and fresh demands on women; a fast-changing perception of the genteel life incorporating greater consumption; difficult conditions for the poor, coupled with higher consumption and educational aspirations, all hint at the gradual shaping of an atmosphere within which the FP propagandists' call for smaller families became intelligible and appealing. The FPP readily appealed to the economic insecurities and aspirations hovering around the home, and the primary responsibility of fathers and mothers towards its maintenance. What then about possible countervailing tendencies, such as for instance, the sentiment around 'United Kerala', or the powerful community politics in Kerala? In other words, while FP was prominently on the state's agenda by the 1960s, how did political society in Kerala react? Indeed, it is well known that these were times when the left hegemony over political society was particularly pronounced, and community politics was also formidable (Mammen 1981; Nossiter 1982). We turn to this question in the next section.[11]

'A People United in Development'

Around the time in which the consumption-oriented family rooted itself in the educated Malayali's vision of the genteel life, the demands for 'United Kerala', to be created by joining together Travancore, Cochin, and Malabar, reached a crescendo. This generally involved a heightened sense of Kerala's singularity within the Indian nation, and vis-à-vis the other cultural unities inhabiting the geographical space of India. The formation of united Kerala was frequently justified as central to preserving the identity of the Malayali people in the Indian nation (Nambiar 1943; Nair 1947; Kurup [1949] 1977; Nair 1951; Gopalan 1954; Thomas 1954; Pillai 1954; Nair 1962). However, this high tide of the perception of Malayali self-interest within the larger totality did not translate itself into pro-natalism, that might have made the task of the family planning publicists more difficult. Indeed, exacerbated sub-nationalism seemed to have demanded a reduction in the number of Malayalis, not an increase.

The same cannot, however, be said about the highly pervasive community-politics characteristic of Malayali society in the 1950s. The view that relegates community organizations in Kerala to the realm of civil society is mistaken indeed: before Independence, communities were powerful players in the field of politics. They were represented in the legislative bodies, and successfully bargained with the state on a range of issues. With national independence, most of them formally announced their withdrawal from the 'political' and claimed the 'socio–economic' as their legitimate space, as if the latter was somehow distanced and preserved in isolation from the former.[12] This was precisely the space of development: community movements proclaimed their commitment to nation-building by promising to actively aid the Indian state in its efforts to transform local society in the image of the modern West, into the Developed Nation.[13] This however scarcely meant that community movements withdrew into civil society. They continued to exercise enormous indirect influence on politics: the politics of numbers had not ceased to be relevant. Most community movements held fast to their role in the 'socio–economic' as representatives of community interests. Pointing to the continuing inequities between various communities, they resisted the interpretation of nationalist sentiment as being fundamentally inimical to community feeling. They vowed to continue to be active to secure for their respective communities the conditions that would ensure them of full citizenship in the projected developed nation of the future.[14] Their political task was to achieve a delicate balance between these two commitments.

In this context, it is hardly surprising that FP often appeared at least ambiguous to advocates of community politics. In a political milieu in which the clout of numbers remained a considerable asset, state-sponsored birth control was easily read as being a step inimical to community interests. From the 1930s onwards, opinion within prominent community movements had been divided about the utility of artificial birth control as an instrument of development. There were many who were convinced that numbers did not matter if the wealth-producing capacities of the community was sufficiently enhanced (for instance, Pillai 1926; Panikar 1930). However, even for those who were convinced of the economic wisdom of reducing numbers, the political reality in which greater numbers did make a difference loomed large. In 1963, the *Malayalarajyam* reiterated an argument against artificial birth control from this vantage-point, already familiar since the 1930s:

> It does not seem that the Catholics in this society will support it ... As for the Ezhavas, they are in general a large community. Ezhava leaders believe that the greatness and advantage of that community lies in their large population.... The Ezhavas and Catholics together form a sizeable portion of the population of Kerala. If these groups do not wholeheartedly participate in population control, what is the utility in the propagation of population control by the Nairs and the Nambutiris? Others will make up for what they reduce. This is because all claims made in Kerala are based on numbers. Such programmes as these will not work until citizens are made into scientifically-oriented, modern-minded individuals. [*Malayalarajyam* 21 December 1963: 2.]

Here, of course, the nation enters. The *Malayalarajyam* endorsed the statement of the minister for Public Health that 'its success [of the Family Planning Programme] lies in viewing it in terms of the national interest.' (p. 2). Successful implementation of FP seemed to require a bridge to be built directly linking the nation and the individual without the intervening particular interests, such as that of the community, interfering. In earlier editorials, the *Malayalarajyam* had explicitly pointed out that the adoption of FP by the Nairs and Nambutiris would be detrimental to their interests, under the present circumstances (13 December 1958: 2; 9 April 1963: 2). Representatives of marginalized social groups, pointing out that numerical strength was the only strength they possessed under current circumstances, had also expressed such doubts.[15] The communists had their own reasons to be suspicious of state-sponsored FP in the 1950s, and these were also reflected in Kerala: for instance, as seen in the arguments of E. Gopalakrishna Menon, the communist member, in the Travancore–Cochin Legislative Assembly, during the debate on the pro-FP resolution introduced by A.P. Udayabhanu in 1951 (*Proceedings of the Travancore-Cochin Legislative Assembly* 1951: 1601–2).

In the 1950s, we find repeated claims made on the strength of numbers, and the reluctance to accept FP often attributed to certain social groups is often readily linked to fear of political decline.[16] The attempt made at Nair–Ezhava unity by Mannath Padmanabhan and R. Sankar in the early 1950s, which aimed at floating a 'Hindu organization' devoid of caste and pitted against Christians and Muslims seems to indicate that the politics of numbers was alive and well, and that it could be easily extended (*Nazrani Deepika* 27 September 1949: 1; 7 November 1949: 2). Those who claimed to have abandoned a political programme were only too eager to prescribe ways of ensuring adequate political representation to their respective communities. In this sense, the scepticism about state-sponsored FP, voiced earlier in the legislative assemblies of Cochin and Travancore was to some extent carried over into the 1950s.[17] In the late 1950s and even in the '60s, the opposition put up by various interest groups and communists was being mentioned as a major hurdle to the success of FP in Kerala.[18]

There is however reason to believe that the fears aired by the *Malayalarajyam* were already, or at least rapidly, becoming redundant in the 1960s. First, there were clear indications that the rifts and fault-lines within communities were deepening, such that 'community-interest' was becoming much more complicated than before (Mammen 1981). Secondly, the entrenchment of 'responsible parenting' and the resultant heightening of domestic burdens seem to have been generally accepted as an emergent reality people had to adjust to. Father Vadakkan, the leading Catholic publicist, remarked about sterilization in an interview that it was a sin, but a thoroughly forgivable one; a necessary evil of sorts:

> Suppose that a father and mother have ten children. Or suppose that there is the fear that the wife might die in childbirth. Or a situation in which one is unable to provide adequate education and food to one's children. I have seen the tears of many such suffering families. If such people accept Family Planning, God will forgive them ... the God who forgave the prostitute Mary Magdalene, the God who forgave thieves and sinners, such a God would certainly forgive the person who submits to the sterilization operation out of sheer misery. [*Kerala Kaumudi* 11 August 1968: 8.]

In the 1930s, communities, especially those less numerous, were acutely alive to the political benefits to be reaped from greater numbers; suggestions to increase numbers without breeding were sometimes contemplated.[19] However, by the 1960s, it was being admitted that with the massive changes in the fundamentals of community, and home life, more children no longer signified the future strength of the community.[20] Redistributionist politics, it appeared, could no longer stall the emergence of conditions under which child rearing appeared increasingly a struggle between meagre resources and multiplying needs. Indeed, it was even being argued that it was not politically wise for the minorities to indulge in 'uncontrolled breeding'—the Muslims were often addressed in these terms (Ali 1967: 4). As for the communists, they had never objected to artificial birth control as a measure of personal choice. In particular contexts, in the 1930s, they emerged as champions of birth control, such as in the Malabar District Board in 1939, in which they passed a resolution demanding that the Madras government open birth control clinics (Jeffrey 2003: 196). In 1957, E.M.S. Nambutiripad clarified the issue in the Kerala State Legislative Assembly that the Communist Party welcomed artificial birth control 'for health reasons', but did not consider it to be a solution 'to the problems facing us today' (*Nazrani Deepika* 20 June 1957: 1). In the communist vision of ideal society, FP figures not so much as an economic instrument as a political one: like the nation, they too needed to clear the political ground so that appeals beyond community loyalties and interests would resonate.[21] Thus, though *Nazrani Deepika* was expressing immense frustration in the communist ministry's considerable interest in FP (pointing out that on this issue, Catholics and communists had generally agreed) (*Nazrani Deepika* 15 April 1958: 2), the interest is not inexplicable.

Given the pervasiveness of the desire for development, it is also possible to understand why the rise of (sub) nationalist sentiment in the 1950s, in the *Aikyakerala* (United Kerala) Movement and outside did not generate any form of pro-natalism. That the widespread propagation of FP seemed to go against the crucial need to actively preserve Kerala's clout in the political game did figure in the discussion on FP in the Travancore–Cochin Legislative Assembly in 1951. Taryattu Kunhittomman, speaking against FP, argued: 'Besides, in the coming days, all our affairs are to be decided through voting. Our representation at the Center is dependent on our population. If so, our population must certainly remain high' (*Proceedings of the Travancore Cochin Legislative Assembly* 1952: 1598). However, such arguments received little elaboration in the course of the 1950s, even with the waxing of the movement for United Kerala.

Not surprisingly, however, as early as the 1930s, a large population, apparently useful in political terms, was admitted to be economically disadvantageous. This was best stated by Kesari A. Balakrishna Pillai, was one of the earliest champions of artificial birth control in Kerala, which he supported on a number of grounds including the economic (Pillai 1989). Nevertheless, writing on the future of the Malayalis in the 1930s, he outlined a situation in which lesser numbers threatened to push them into a peripheral position within the forthcoming Indian nation. The way out, it was clarified, was the vigorous pursuit of accumulation through development:

> People fewer in numbers may gain an important place in ruling their motherland and in other affairs by developing their abilities in other matters. But Malayalis seem to possess no such advantage in comparison with other peoples. Economically and industrially, the Malayali's position, when compared to that of others, is very backward.... There is the possibility that in the independent India of the future, Malayalis may become an insignificant minority and gradually decline, becoming slaves to other

peoples. This terrible future is not because Nature has been unfavourable... [Pillai 1934: 24–5.]

Pillai's advice was that Malayalis should rapidly modernize all modes of life-sustenance, and multiply the means of wealth creation. Wealth-creation, however, seemed to require less population pressure on land. By the end of the 1940s, these ideas had gained considerable circulation among the modern-educated in Kerala, through a variety of sites ranging from textbooks to the conferences of community movements. By the 1950s, the necessity of large-scale industry which required large amounts of capital accumulation was being urgently pressed in public discussion, and the implications of this for Kerala's relation with the central government were clearly drawn out. E.M.S. Nambutiripad, writing on Kerala's economic problems in 1956, pointed out that the goal of development could not be achieved without the active support of the central government, and active cooperation with it in large-scale developmental activities. He wrote:

> This task, however, cannot be carried out by the State of Kerala—its people and its government—by themselves. [This is so] precisely because Kerala is not an independent country but an integral part of India; our economy is not an isolated one but part of the general economy spread throughout India.... So we Malayalis can finds solutions to our problems only as part of the organized efforts carried out by the people and the government all over India to reform and develop India's economy. [Nambutiripad 1956: 7.]

EMS stated unambiguously that the way out of Kerala's economic ills lay in 'An all-India economic plan that will help in the speedy growth of large-scale industry, the reform of agriculture based on this and improve trade, industry and transport. Only when problems are solved in an all-India basis will Kerala's problems be solved' (p. 53). The FPP seemed efficacious in that it could help to create the crucial condition for wealth-creation mentioned: lower population pressure on land, and on the resources of the government, which would have to otherwise devote quite a large share to social development. Speaking on radio in support of FPP, E.M.S. Nambutiripad stressed precisely this point (reported in *Matrubhumi* 21 September 1967: 3). No wonder then that many who enthusiastically embraced it also endorsed the unity and self-assertion of Malayalis as a people within the Indian subcontinent. Indeed, the Kerala-of-the-future was definitely imagined in terms of linguistic unity and a unique cultural identity; but equally, it was imagined in terms of development. In an evocative vision of the Kerala-of-the-future, E.M.S. Nambutiripad conjures up the vision of a people united in development, upon whom the scientific temper is regnant, whose modes of life-sustenance are thoroughly modernized. He calls this society the *Mavelinadu* of the future, referring to the mythical kingdom celebrated in Malayali myths, in which no one knew any want, treachery, or misery (Nambutiripad [1946b] 1999: 288–347). This new Kerala was to be thickly populated with large-scale industries, scientifically-managed farms, hydel plants; and this was pointed to as the ideal environment in which 'freedom', defined as 'being able to live without servility to another and with universal access to food and other basic needs of life ...' was promised as the means to thrive (p. 344). Once the desire for such a Kerala, which obviously required massive mobilization of resources, was set in place; Malayali self-assertion and identity became perfectly compatible with the call for a reduction in their numbers as urgently as possible. It is also quite evident that 'responsible parenting' fitted well within this vision, directing people more into the business of shaping productive human forces in the home.[22]

Notes

1 It may also be noted that the descriptions of crisis in matrilineal joint families in many of these autobiographies often highlight as causes not 'unnatural' marriage practices, but rather the intense economic pressures of the early twentieth century, and the coming of new individual and family values. See for instance, Cherukad Govinda Pisharady, *Jeevitappata*, Thiruvananthapuram, Deshabhimani Books, 1984; K. Kannan Nair, Kozhikode, *Atmakatha*, Matrubhumi, 1989, and V.R. Parameshwaran Pillai, *Aa Ezhupatu Varshangal*, Thiruvananthapuram, 1974.

2 This does not mean that the guru did not approve of modern marriage. In a message to the SNDP Yogam in 1909, he clearly approved of a legal provision

giving a portion of the individual earnings of the husband to the wedded wife and their children. Quoted in Meera Velayudhan, 'Reform, Law and Gendered Identity', *in* M.A. Oommen (ed.), *Kerala's Development Experience,* vol. I, New Delhi, ISS and Concept Publishers, 1999, 64.

[3] Interestingly, the focus on transforming fatherhood to facilitate the entry of the state into the family is still an important strategy of family planning programmes in the third world. Writing on the family planning programme television advertisements in Egypt, Kamran Ali points out that the state is attempting to create a 'new kind of patriarch ... [who is] responsible about his civil duties and subservient to the state; duties that include enabling the state to have access to female bodies for contraceptive purposes without hindrance from male partners'. Kamran Asdar Ali, 'Myths, Lies and Impotence: Structural Adjustment and Male Voice in Egypt', *Comparative Studies of South Asia, Africa and the Middle-East*, 23,1, 2003, 327.

[4] The critic Tayattu Sankaran has noted that her conception of the child differs significantly from earlier notions of the child that celebrate it as a source of joy, in that it sees the child as the nucleus of the mature human being, the responsibility for which lies with the mother who must nurture it. Tayattu Sankaran, 'Bharateeyata', in *Balamani Amma Sashtipoorthy Smaranika*, Kozhikode, 1969, 65–6.

[5] See his speech at a Nair meeting at Mavelikkara, in which he argued that men and women who had more than two children were deserving of punishment. *Malayala Manorama,* 19 Aug. 1963, 4; speech at Ambalappuzha, *Malayala Rajyam* 3 Oct. 1964, 1; speech at Pattanapuram, *Malayala Manorama,* 30 Nov. 1961, 4.

[6] Interestingly, while we do find such emphasis on the transformation of the family as a fundamental condition for the rooting of the modern state in other colonial societies, the emphasis on gender roles is not always the same. The May Fourth Movement (1919) in China, for instance, strongly upheld a eugenics-influenced view of social transformation, in which considerable importance was conceded to birth control. Even so, the imagining of male–female familial roles here is quite striking in its stress on the couple's sharing of domestic responsibilities. See Hiroko Sakamoto, 'The Cult of "Love and Eugenics" in May Fourth Movement Discourse', *Positions: East Asia Cultures Critique* 12, 2, 2004, 329–76.

[7] The Nayadis were certainly neither parasites nor 'useless'; these characterizations owe a lot to the colonial representations of nomadic people. They were often thought to be skilled thieves, stealing agricultural produce, but their skills in catching rodents, which they consumed, were also valued, as late as the 1960s. Farmers often allowed them into their fields and gardens in return for their catching rodent pests that devastated crops.

[8] In Kerala's powerful literary public sphere, the criticism of the Malayali's dependence on salaried work was far more powerful. The optimism exuded by early Malayalam novels about the value of employment in family-centred political

struggles is almost completely extinguished in mid-twentieth century modern Malayalam literature. Salaried employment does not appear so liberating now: increasingly bleak portrayals of the individual caught between a poverty-stricken and oppressive traditional society, and the equally or more alienating cog-like existence of the employee in modern bureaucracy, army, or business, figure. (See, for instance, E.V. Ramakrishnan, 'Pattalakathakalile Rashtrasankalpam' (The concept of the nation in army stories), in *Vakkile Samooham*, Kottayam, D.C. Books, 1997, 41–9) in which the disillusionment with the post-colonial state in the 'army' stories of writers like Nandanar, Kovilan, and Parappuram is discussed). Employment begins to appear to be an inevitability into which the Malayali is pushed, but without which survival would be impossible.

[9] Indeed, the changes that had begun to be conspicuous in everyday consumption were already noticed in the early part of the century. For an argument that linked consumption, changing lifestyles, and women's incomes, see Pennamma Bhayi, 'Our Economic Position and Women', in J. Devika (ed.), *Her-self Early Writings on Gender by Malayalee Women,* Kolkata, Stree, 2005, 154–57.

[10] See, for instance, M.O. Joseph, 'Janananiyantrana Prasthanam' (The birth control movement), *Nazrani Deepika,* 22 Dec. 1933, 8; Jose Vakayil Parambil, 'Janananiyantranam' (Birth control), *Deepika Weekly,* 5, 46, 1952, 17–19; 'Lokalokam' (editor's column on world affairs), *Swajanaranjini,* 1, 2, 1934, 33–41; 'Sanatananiyantranam' (Birth control), *Aryakeralam,* 1,1, 1936, 3–6.

[11] The significance of this should not be underestimated. As Agnes Reidman has pointed out in the case of family planning work in Nigeria, notions such as 'excess number of children' or 'unmet need for FP services' have very different resonances when they form part of questions addressed to different social institutions. For instance, when children are perceived to belong to, and to be the responsibility of as much the lineage as of the parents, such questions may elicit very different answers. See Agnes Reidmann, *Science that Colonizes: A Critique of Fertility Studies in Africa*, Philadelphia, Temple University Press, 1993, 69–78.

[12] See Joseph Naduvattumuri, speech at Latin Christian Mahajanasabha Annual Conference at Thiruvananthapuram, *Nazrani Deepika*, 13 May 1949, 1; Joseph Maliakkal, 'Catholica Conference: Oru Tiruttal' (Catholic Conference: a clarification), *Nazrani Deepika*, 15 June 1949, 3. Sections of the Travancore Muslim League also announced the renunciation of their political programme in 1949, though it was strongly opposed by others: see, Jamal, *Kunhusahib* (A biography of the Muslim leader P.K. Kunhu), Kochi, 1975, 175. In an editorial in 1961, *Kerala Kaumudi* discussed the implications of such renunciation, arguing that community politics was unavoidable, but tolerable only because almost all community movements had agreed to remain 'non-political'. See 'Vargeeyatayum Mukhyamantrimarute Sammelanavum' (Communal politics and the Chief Ministers' conference), *Kerala Kaumudi,* 15 Aug. 1961, 2.

[13] Indeed, it was even argued that the politics of redistribution was taking too

much space, and in the conferences and meetings of community movements they were urged to pay attention to the task of nation building and developmental activities. Endorsing the exhortation of the Travancore–Kochi Joint Nair Conference in 1947 that community movements should focus on developmental activities, *Nazrani Deepika* wrote: 'Community organisations have long concentrated on political affairs. Although political programmes have been abandoned now, many community movements continue to focus on political affairs. They are not seen to be displaying this interest and energy shown in political matters, in economic programmes.' 'Samudayasanghatanakal' (Community movements), *Nazrani Deepika,* 14 Sept. 1949, 2. Also see, speech by Paliath P.K.P. Achan, *Nazrani Deepika* 13 Sept. 1949, 3. Almost all the speeches of Mannath Padmanabhan in the 1950s and '60s uphold this point without, however, sacrificing the communal viewpoint. See his speeches in Kidangoor A.N. Gopalakrishna Pillai (ed.), *Mannathinte Sampoorna Kritikal,* Kottayam, Vidyarthimitram Publishers, 1977.

14 See, speech, Manmadhan Nair, *Nazrani Deepika,* 13 Sept. 1949, 3; speech by Seeti Sahib, 'Vargeeyatayum Desheeyatvavum' (Communalism and nationalism) [1958] in Abu Siddique, *Seethi Sahib: Jeevacharitram,* Kozhikode, 1966, 208–15; statement by Joseph Chazhikkad, *Nazrani Deepika,* 5 May 1949; speech, P.K. Sukumaran, *Kerala Kaumudi,* 15 Nov. 1967, 2; editorial, 'SNDP Yogam', *Kerala Kaumudi* 16 Dec. 1970, 2.

15 See speech by T.A. Kunhumaideen Kunhu, Travancore–Cochin Legislative Assembly, Third Session 3 April 1951, *Proceedings of the Travancore–Cochin Legislative Assembly,* vol. iii nos. I& II, Government of Travancore–Cochin, Thiruvananthapuram, 1952, 1605–6. Also, speech by P.C. Adichan (who represented the depressed classes in the Travancore–Cochin Legislative Assembly), in which he pointed out that encouraging people of the scheduled castes and tribes to take to birth control would negatively affect their political interests, as reservations were promised only for a decade. *Nazrani Deepika,* 29 Sept. 1951, 3.

16 Innumerable instances may be cited here. To mention just a few: editorial, *Nazrani Deepika* 27 Sept. 1949, 2; Editorial, *Nazrani Deepika,* 29 June: 1949; Speech by Mannath Padmanabhan and R. Sankar at the Pattanamtitta Hindu Conference, *Nazrani Deepika,* 15 Feb. 1950, 6; report of resolution of the SNDP director board, *Malayala Manorama,* 29 Sept. 1961, 4; speech by Mannath Padmanabhan, *Matrubhumi,* 19 Feb. 1964, 3. Interestingly, in this speech he argued that the fight for a fair share of resources and openings for Nairs should not interfere with their commitment to FP.

17 In 1950, Kunhuraman, Minister in the Travancore–Cochin Cabinet denied in the Legislative Assembly that the government had plans to support FP, saying that the government did not believe the population was excessive (*Nazrani Deepika,* 12 Nov. 1950, 3); in 1951 too, no effort from the government's side was admitted to in response to similar questions (Answer to Question no. 632,

17 March 1951, Third Session, *Proceedings of the Travancre–Cochin Legislative Assembly,* vol. iii, i, and ii, Government of Travancore–Cochin, Thiruvananthapuram, 1952, 584–5; report in *Nazrani Deepika* (7 November 1952, 2) on question raised in Travancore–Cochin Legislative Assembly on whether an FP clinic had been opened in Travancore to which the health minister V. Madhavan replied that the government had no plans to support FP; In 1953, in reply to the suggestion that FP work should be added on to the Kuttanad Social Development Project, the Travanocre–Cochin chief minister A.J. John clarified that it would not be so (*Nazrani Deepika,* 7 Sept. 1953: 1); even when governmental initiative was conceded, it was with considerable qualification. See, for instance, report of question by V. Shreedharan in the Travancore–Cochin Legislative Assembly, *Nazrani Deepika,* 19 Oct. 1955, 3; report of question to minister P.K. Kunhu to which he replied that the FPP was the Centre's interest, and not that of his party (*Nazrani Deepika,* 21 July 1954, 5). Even in 1970, the question of whether FP would not upset the balance between communities was being raised in the Kerala State Legislature. See, report, *Kerala Kaumudi,* 30 Jan. 1970, 5.

[18] See answer to starred question no. 846 by R. Prakasham to health minister Dr A.R. Menon, 30 March 1959, *Proceedings of the Kerala Legislative Assembly,* vol. vii, 25–36, 1960, 2396–7; statement by A.R.Menon, *Nazrani Deepika,* 5 July 1957, 3; editorial, *Matrubhumi,* 14 Feb. 1967, 3; Dr C.O. Karunakaran, 'Kutumbasamvidhanam Avidayum Ividayum' (Family Planning, there and here), *Kerala Kaumudi,* 18 May 1968, 2.

[19] See Ambady Narayani Pothuvalsyar, 'Ambalavasi Samudayam' (The Ambalavasi community), *Yuvachaitanyam,* 1, 1, Oct.–Nov. 1933, 46–7; K.V. Sankara Warrier, 'Samudaya Parishkaranam—Ekeekaranam' (Community reform—unification), *Swajanaranjini,* 1, 4, 1934, 132–6; *Nambutiri Family Regulation Committee Report,* Yogakshemam, Thrissur, 1925, 42–3. For an account of the intense efforts to unite the coastal communities into the 'Dheevara' community, see Ettumanoor Gopalan, *Dewer Enna Karmadheeran,* Kochi, Dewer Smaraka Samiti, 1993. The Nair Conference held at Mavelikkara in 1932 passed a resolution relating to increasing their numbers by amalgamating sub-castes (*The Mahila* 12, 4/5, 1932, 160–1). The Ezhavas, apparently, had already begun this process, see N.K. Damodaran, 'Parishuddha Ezhavan, Chettatta Ezhavan', *Kerala Kaumudi,* 4 Aug. 1968, 4.

[20] See, for instance, articles in the *Souvenir of the Kerala Catholic Regional Seminar,* Dec. 1969.

[21] Communist authors advocated a strategic approach towards community movements that would steer them towards development, perceived to have homogenizing qualities. See, for instance, E.M.S. Nambutiripad, 'Keralattile Samudayasanghatanakal: Avayodu Perumarendatengane?' (Community movements in Kerala: how to approach them?), *Matrubhumi,* 25 July 1936 (rept. *in* P. Govinda Pillai (ed.), *EMS Sampoornakritikal,* vol. 2,

Thiruvananthapuram, Chinta, 1999, 86–94; E.M.S. Nambutiripad, 'Nambutiriye Manushyanakkan' (To make the Malayala brahmin human), Kozhikode, Deshabhimani, 1945; Kambissery Karunakaran, 'Communisavum Communalisavum' (Communism and communalism), *Prabhatam,* 1, 8, Jan. 1945, 1,12.

22 The connection between rising consumption, modern education, and the adoption of the small family norm has now been widely noticed around the world (Jack Goody, 'Globalisation, Population and Ecology', paper presented at the International Conference on Theoretical Topics in Ecological Economics, Trieste, Italy, 10–12 Feb. 2003), and in other historical periods (Gloria L. Main, 'Rocking the Cradle: Downsizing the New England Family', *Journal of Interdisciplinary History,* 37, 1, 2006, 35–58). However, I want to conclude this chapter by pointing out that in societies where 'developmental idealism' has not yet developed roots, this change is not often celebrated. This of course does not mean that these societies have rejected contraception. Indeed, as Elise Levin notes in Guinea, though the older women deeply lament the 'changes that made large families difficult to support, they were quick to use the new contraceptives to their advantage' (Elise C. Levin, 'Women's Childbearing Decisions in Guinea: Life Course Perspectives and Historical Change', *Africa Today,* 47, 3/4, 2000, 79). While individuals do accept birth limitation as inevitable in the context of economic difficulty, they also admit that the straightened circumstances that make the existence of communal life precarious also drive them to the FP clinic (Pamela Feldman-Savelsberg, *Plundered Kitchens, Empty Wombs: Threatened Reproduction and Identity in the Cameroon Grassfields,* Ann Arbor, University of Michigan Press, 1999).

3

Disenfranchisement, Development and Family Planning

The Importance of Failure

In the earlier chapters I attempted to argue that FP became acceptable in Malayali society when it was established as (a) a practice that would promote sexual self-discipline among individuals rather than undermine it, and (b) a practice that would help realize the new ideals of family and the gendered roles inscribed in them, under changing and difficult material circumstances. In this chapter, I would like to demonstrate how FP gained acceptance too as a practice that was projected as holding the potential to help Malayalis tide over their economic disenfranchisement within the Indian nation, widely felt in the 1960s. In the discussions that projected FP as the solution to Kerala's ills, the Malayali reading public was steadfastly directed towards the wisdom and necessity of FP not only as 'responsible parents' or 'sexually disciplined individuals', but also as the patriotic citizens of a (sub-)nationality.[1] Severe anxieties about (sub-)national identity and delayed economic take-off in the 1960s formed a crucial backdrop against which FP was presented cogently in Kerala as a practical instrument of development. Indeed, the arguments raised in favour of improving the quality of life of the people through FP were themselves pegged to the desire for robust economic growth.

The term 'disenfranchisement' has been relatively recently coined in the context of global governance issues to 'reflect the limitations of social actors when they try to engage with international regimes for sustainable development ... [It refers to] [B]eing deprived of the capability to participate and influence agenda-setting and decision-making in international regimes for sustainable development' (Fischer and Green 2004: 66, 68). These authors further refine the term by pointing out that disenfranchisement does not imply the absence of the disenfranchised from formal bodies; they may indeed enjoy equal legal standing with others in formal bodies. Actually it is often the lack of ability to effectively intervene in decision-making processes despite a formal presence in decision-making bodies and this is what the authors call 'disenfranchisement' when they talk of nation-states in international bodies. I find this term particularly useful to characterize a dominant mood in the Malayali public of the 1960s: 'a sense of being disenfranchised' within the nation-state was certainly pronounced in Malayali public discussions in the 1960s.

In other words, I contend that the FPP in Kerala gained substantial momentum in the particularly difficult decade of the 1960s, in which the (sub-)national pride of the Malayalis was being offended in many ways. As was argued towards the end of chapter two, developmentalism occupied an extraordinary centrality in mid-twentieth century projections of the Kerala-of-the future. As mentioned there, in this vision, larger numbers were not at all necessary for a prosperous (sub-)national future. By the late 1950s, less optimistic predictions regarding Kerala's economic growth made FP appear no less than an absolute necessity for the state. The suspicion that developmental interventions in Kerala were being throttled both by external foes and internal constraints began to be frequently articulated, reaching a feverish pitch in the 1960s, even touching the already raw nerve of (sub-) national pride. The food crisis of the 1960s was acutely felt, Kerala being a food-deficient state, and this heightened the sense of dependency of the Malayalis, and their ire against the central government. Complaints about the neglect of Kerala in large-scale industrialization continued to be voiced in the 1960s with renewed indignation. Prospects of migration seemed to be rapidly dwindling, especially with anti-immigrant riots in Mumbai. The various options, which had been advanced earlier as solutions to the 'population problem', seemed inaccessible for many reasons, not least of which was the marginality of the Malayali people vis-à-vis the Indian state. Under such difficult conditions, it became quite easy to project population reduction as a panacea to the developmental afflictions of Kerala; as a kind of immediate step to resolve the 'population problem', now readily identified as the root cause of Kerala's lack of growth, and by implication, its inability to assert itself within the Indian nation.

The intense anxieties in the north over differential population growth between the north and south in the twentieth century have been extensively commented upon (Teitelbaum and Winter 1985: 50; Donaldson 1990; Szreter 1993: 663; Symonds and Carder 1996). The importance of the global context is evident when we see that in the earlier decades, birth control was only one among many solutions proposed for the amelioration of the 'population problem' in Kerala. However, since the late-1950s, the importance granted to FP began to grow. This shift roughly coincides with the mid-twentieth century shift in the discourse of population and development in the first world. In the 1940s and early 1950s, it was argued that the 'population problem' of the south could be resolved through developmental intervention in production, such as rapid industrialization (for instance, Davis 1951: 229). By roughly the mid-1950s and subsequently, population growth was seen to be overwhelming developmental efforts, and serious theoretical work sought to confirm this linkage (Coale and Hoover 1958). The first-world-centred shifts within the Indian national policy on birth control and health have also been well-charted by now (Myrdal 1968: 2151–64; Banerji 1971; Qadeer 1998); so also is the crisis of Nehruvian developmentalism in the mid-1960s (Deshpande 1993). However, it is my burden in this chapter to show that the local context is also of equal importance in building a case for the utility of FP as an instrument of state planning, for the successful projection of population reduction as an important condition for growth. I wish to stress how important some local *failures* were in forging a public atmosphere here conducive to FP. The usual practice in academic and non-academic writings on the subject has been to emphasize local achievements or 'advantages' (like the widespread induction of women into modern family values, mores, and aspirations—thinly veiled under confusing usages like 'female literacy/education').

This chapter draws upon the extensive discussions on population as a problem in development in the Malayali public sphere in the mid-twentieth century. The aspirations of (sub-)national economic self-sufficiency through accelerated development, and the projection of FP as an important means to realize this, circulated among a substantial and growing reading public familiar with the vocabulary of development. Again, this is not to discount the fact that the FP propaganda did significantly highlight the argument that limiting fertility held considerable personal/familial gains for individuals. However, a broad consensus on the general utility of FP's utility for the society as a whole, and in the long run, did help justify the government's assumption of the role of the primary provider of FP services in Kerala in a dynamic and commanding sense.

The first section focuses upon explication of the 'population problem' in the public debates in Malayali society in a period spanning roughly from the 1930s to the 1950s, to see how, and to what degree was birth control recognized as a solution to it. The next section follows this discussion into the post-Independence period to see how the stage is set for the projection of FP as a major answer to the vexed question of lagging economic growth in Kerala. In the last section, the effort is to position the successful promotion of the FPP within the histories of developmentalism, and civil social activism in Kerala.

Pathogenic Numbers?

> Burgeoning population is the most critical problem plaguing Kerala, which has earned the notoriety of being a problem state. The steadily increasing population is at the root of all the vexing problems facing the State... One can well guess how food availability and other conditions of life will end up if the population continues to increase at this rate. [*Kerala Kaumudi* 30 June 1967: 2.]

Vociferously arguing in favour of a vigorous FPP in the 1960s, Malayali newspapers were seeking to convince their readership that the maladies seen to be infecting Malayali society had sprung from their inordinately large numbers. Also, a consensus seemed to have been reached on the utility of birth control as an economic measure central to the eventual goal of all participants, of economic growth.

This consensus, however, was not some automatic or naturally forthcoming response. It was forged in and through several contexts of discussion around matters relating to economic growth and development ever since the early decades of the twentieth century in the Malayali public sphere. In each of these, 'large population' came to figure as a major cause, often the single most conspicuous cause, of the malaise being discussed, and at times, artificial birth control was proposed as a possible solution. However, in the early phases of these discussions—in the early decades of the twentieth century—it was granted relatively minor importance among the several solutions that were advanced. By the mid-twentieth century, however, this scene seemed to be rapidly changing: population regulation through the popularization of artificial birth control was granted a place alongside large-scale industrialization or intensive agriculture as a developmental measure. In this section I briefly consider some of these discussions in their early phases, so that the contours of the transformation are more evident.

In Travancore, the serious food deficit was a matter of discussion in the Malayalam press from at least the second decade of the twentieth century. Three features of these discussions are worth noting for our purposes. First, the importance granted to population pressure did not mean that other factors were underplayed. For example, many authors acknowledged the effects of the integration of Travancore into the world economy by the mid-nineteenth century on food production. Secondly, the importance that was conceded to the large population in generating food deficit did not automatically foreground population regulation by the state as a developmental solution; rather, a multiplicity of solutions was proposed. Thirdly, powerful voices questioned the close and necessary association assumed between low food production and high population, and the sagacity of birth control to increase production itself.

To elaborate on the first point mentioned above: Ward and Conner, surveying Travancore in the early nineteenth century, found that it was producing enough grain to meet its demands. About 30 per cent of the land under cultivation in Travancore were rice lands, along with another 45 per cent devoted to temporary cultivation of rice and other grains on hill slopes. This began to alter in the latter half of the nineteenth century, and paddy imports began to rise, reaching a level of 45 per cent of all imports by 1913–14 (Rammohan 1996: 64–5). A major backdrop for this was the gradual extinction of hill-paddy cultivation or *malamkrishi* with the arrival of the metropolitan planters (Rammohan 1996: 68–9). At the same time, food requirements were hiked by various factors such as 'the influx of people from the Tamil country seeking work in the plantations, increase in the total as well as share of population not engaged in the production of food crops—they were engaged in industry and plantations—and increase in purchasing power of certain sections of the people' (Rammohan 1996: 70). Though probably more visible in hindsight, this, however, was not entirely missed by contemporary commentators. In several newspaper articles as well as in speeches on the topic in the 1930s and 1940s, Travancore's increasing population was identified as a major reason for the insufficiency of food production.[2] Nevertheless, the effects of the integration of Travancore into the world economy in the mid-nineteenth century were often remarked upon as equally crucial. A prominent commentator, G. Raman Menon, remarked thus in the late 1920s about the food deficit:

> About fifty or sixty years back people in Travancore used to be amply fed by the rice produced here itself. In those days, rice or paddy was not imported from Burma. That was not needed. Even just about twenty-five years ago, plenty of paddy used to be brought down from the hills and sold in the lakeside and the seaside. Nowadays, those who live in the hill areas subsist on Burma rice.... The larger part of the best hill lands have been either

> leased out to European capitalists or made into reserve forests, this is the reason why hill-paddy cultivation has become extinct. [Menon, G. Raman 1929: 1]

Several observers repeatedly pointed out the danger entailed by excessive promotion of cash crop cultivation. In 1941, the *Nazrani Deepika* bluntly reminded its readers that humans could not eat rubber, and so the neglect of food crops was unforgivable (22 February 1941: 4); by then this was a familiar refrain that ran through much of the thinking on agriculture in Travancore and Cochin. Throughout the 1920s, '30s and '40s, several authors and speakers stressed the necessity of granting hill lands to the poor for the cultivation of food crops in order to ward off mass poverty. Often they pointed in vociferous terms to the unfair advantage granted to planters. In one of its editorials, the *Nazrani Deepika* demanded that the landless poor of all communities must be given land in the hill areas. The conservation argument was rejected on the grounds that it was frequently relaxed for the plantations (28 June 1939: 2). Kannan Devan Company was given 1,17,588 acres of first-grade forestland, and Brooke Bond would have secured similar concessions from the dewan in 1926, but the Regent Maharani of Travancore and the Travancore Legislative Assembly opposed it (Kooiman 1995: 36). It was also recognized that the loss of the fertility of the soil and the fragmentation of agricultural land were being brought about by reasons other than that of high population pressure alone (Rammohan 1996: 110; *ND* 2 April 1941: 2). It is also worth remarking that similar, if more serious, problems were identified in Malabar during roughly the same period: population density was identified to be a major hurdle in the Malabar Tenancy Report of 1940 (cited in Kunhikrishnan 1996: 85). The anthropologist Adrian Mayer, doing fieldwork in Malabar in the early 1950s, made similar observations (Mayer 1952: 129–30; 150). An editorial in the 1950s citing a memorandum submitted by the members of parliament from Malabar to the prime minister on Malabar's problems, listed unemployment, lack of capital, food deficit and population density (*Matrubhumi* 8 October 1955: 5).

Besides, a variety of solutions were being proposed, and this included migration to less-populated lands, a change in diet, and intensive agriculture. These were to appear far more frequently by the late 1940s, '50s, and well into the '60s, when they were proposed along with FP as part of a composite solution to the food crisis, which include several suggestions such as intensive and extensive agriculture, industrialization, and migration.[3] In 1951, A.P. Udayabhanu suggested a change in Malayali rice-based diet (*Proceedings of the Travancore–Cochin Legislative Assembly* 1952: 1653). Later, the first communist ministry in Kerala tried to popularize macaroni made from tapioca flour, which failed to catch on. Periodical attempts to convince Malayalis of the need to change their diet continued (Nambutiripad [1944] 2000: 82; *Matrubhumi* 29 June 1962: 6; *Kerala Kaumudi* 12 May 1967: 2). Help from the central government in obtaining food grains was suggested at an early stage. The dewan of Travancore, Sir C.P. Ramaswamy Aiyar, speaking in 1944 on Travancore's food-crisis, pointed out that it could have been readily eased if greater central direction of the movement of foodstuffs, so that they reached deficit areas effectively, had been operative (Aiyar [1944] 1945: 263). Later, it was repeatedly argued that the Centre did have an obligation to help, as it was making massive gains from Kerala's cash-crop exports (Oommen 1963). As E.M.S. Nambutiripad expressed it in 1953, the hope was that 'many of our products are important items in India's foreign exports, and so Kerala has an important place in the Indian economy itself. We can use this [advantage] to compel other states and the Centre to provide us with enough food.' (Nambutiripad [1953] 2000: 317–18). This argument was frequently advanced in the 1960s, especially in the context of the massive food crisis. The reflections of the Gandhians and the Sarvodaya activists of these decades on the food deficit, which upfronted the responsibility of the local community to provide food to all its members, and envisaged the reorganization of production accordingly, were also audible.[4] So also was the argument that transferring the ownership of land to the cultivator could be the most effective way of enhancing agricultural yield. Thus the admission of the problem of increasing numbers by these texts did not directly foreground population control as the way out of the problem of food deficit.

Thirdly, scepticism about linking rising numbers and poor food productivity in these times was not negligible. Publicists like P.J. Thomas, Puttezhattu Raman Menon, and P.K. Sukumaran, who stayed well within developmentalist thinking in their reflections on the food deficit (though with distinctly different political shades to their brands of developmentalism), directly opposed the population thesis in several speeches and articles.[5] P.J. Thomas, for instance, strongly argued way back in the 1930s and well into the 1950s, that a large workforce must be considered an asset rather than a liability. Addressing the Ernakulam Village Uplift Conference in 1939, he declared that the problem was the underutilization of the available labour force, and not the spurt in numbers (*ND* 1 February 1939: 2). In fact, he pointed out in 1951, while discussing the effects of the fall in the rate of increase of population in Minachil *taluk* of Kottayam district, that such a decline need not necessarily trigger an improvement in agricultural productivity. Indeed, the reverse could well result. The fall was largely due to the migration of farming families to Malabar seeking land, and this, he reminds, is not conducive to the betterment of agriculture (*ND* 4 May 1951: 1). Other authors were making such arguments by the 1930s (for instance, Pillai 1936: 132–3). Generally, the optimism regarding the power of science and technology, accompanied by efficient planning and management of production and distribution, to increase yields, provide gainful livelihoods is manifest in many such texts. In others, Puttezhattu Raman Menon's writings, for instance, the excessive place granted to market-driven agriculture to the detriment of local needs is sharply criticized. In Malabar, the communist Kisan Sangham faced the food crisis of the 1940s not only by campaigning for intensive cultivation and for extensive cultivation—often by pressurizing the landlords, but also by maintaining vigilance against black-marketing and improving the public distribution system (Kunhikrishnan 1996). Nevertheless, as we shall see, by the late 1950s, population control came to be increasingly recognized as an important component of the efforts to resolve the food crisis. More usually than not, it was projected as one element of a 'composite recommendation' of which the other components were often intensified agriculture, industrialization, migration, and changes in food habits. However, it was also observed that FP was perhaps the most immediately practical of all the options. How this came to be will be discussed later.

A second context of discussion in which population regulation appeared as an important solution was around unemployment. Here, again, the growth in population was soon identified as a major cause, and population management had been proposed among the solutions quite early. The *Report of the Unemployment Enquiry Committee* in Travancore (1928) considered the hypothesis that overpopulation may be a cause of unemployment here. Yet it made a somewhat qualified point on the matter. Claiming that the 'state of overpopulation exists when the numbers of the people may be such as to press upon the means of subsistence, i.e., when its rate of increase is higher than its rate of productivity' (p. 40), it examined the relevant figures to arrive at the conclusion that 'the state is overpopulated under the existing economic considerations'. (p. 42). It observed that economic modernization in Travancore was certainly not a duplication of the situation in Europe during the Industrial Revolution when the growing population was absorbed by the expanding economy, and that population growth did not bode well for Travancore (p. 44). A few of the witnesses examined by the Committee had suggested popularization of various direct and indirect means of birth control, but public opinion was not inclined to this. The authors of the report recognized the limited nature of the economic modernization of Travancore, and birth control was projected as relevant *in that context.* While this gloomy inevitability would be driven home persistently in the media by the 1960s, many writers and speakers were more optimistic in the early years. In 1939, P.J. Thomas pointed out that unemployment was surmountable if labour power was rationally utilized, and that

> the world's best market lies at the doorstep of Cochin. India with its forty-crore population is the largest area of free commerce in the world. States like

> Cochin, Travancore and Mysore, which have gained economic progress, can transform this vast market to their advantage if they organize their production and marketing judiciously. [*ND* 1 February 1939: 2.]

In the Travancore–Cochin Legislative Assembly, P. Balakrishnan Thampi initiated a discussion on 'excess manpower in the State', which he remarked was 'both its strength as well as its weakness', and that effective state intervention could turn it into an asset. He recommended that the central government should be asked to consider people from Travancore–Cochin for the defence and other central government services; that migration to thinly-populated regions of India should be encouraged; and that labour should be conscripted for building public works (*Proceedings of the Travancore–Cochin Assembly* 1951: 1209). In the 1950s, leftist thinking on unemployment was characterized by the same optimism. C. Unny Raja, a prominent communist intellectual, writing in 1956, echoed much the same confidence. He remarked that that the high population density was increasing the pressure on land, and recommended rapid industrialization as the solution to unemployment (Raja 1956). Differences of opinion largely centred on the specific form of industrialization required: it was pointed out, for instance, that natural resources should be utilized in a way that generated maximum employment. P.J. Thomas, for example, pointed out in 1952 that the recently established industries in Travancore–Cochin, such as aluminum, glass, and rayon largely brought raw materials from outside the state, eyeing the cheap electricity, and did not employ much labour. 'Only if small industries that employ large numbers and utilize natural resources abundantly obtained in the state are established in various places will the people of this populous state benefit' (*ND* 31 July 1952: 2). Another solution proposed was migration. In 1958, P.J. Thomas strongly opposed those who prescribed birth control as a solution to the ills of Kerala, claiming that a reduction of the Malayali population would negatively impact the Indian nation:

> only very few areas of the world have seen such vigorous activities to make the earth productive as in Kerala. Where else in India have such activities as turning an unproductive lake into grain-bearing fields, and transforming

> densely forested hill areas into garden land bearing gold, been undertaken to the extent as they have been in Kerala? ... People who are capable of such creative labour ought not to be reduced through birth control and other means, but rehabilitated to other parts of India and abroad for the sake of economic progress ... [*ND* 15 August 1953: 2.]

Yet by the end of the 1950s it seemed as though population regulation needed to be considered as a developmental measure. As in the case of the discussion on the food deficit, here too, when organized population control was suggested, it almost inevitably appeared to be part of a 'composite solution' (for instance, Tharakan 1956: 100–20). Dr P.S. Lokanathan's *Industrial Survey Report* (1962), much discussed in the press in the early 1960s, upheld the necessity of a multi-pronged approach, including accelerated industrialization, technological upgradation, intensified food crop production, and population regulation (*MM* 1 May 1962: 2).

A third context of discussion in which population growth emerged as a major explanation was that of the massive 'beggar problem' that arose in the wake of the terrible destitution brought about by the economic effects of the Second World War (Jeffrey 2003: 196). Nevertheless, the discussion largely focused on the management of the hungry and homeless streaming into towns as beggars. The *Report of the Beggar Relief Committee* of the state of Cochin (1944), for example, cited the pressure of population along with the decline of joint families and unemployment as one of the major reasons for the growth of mendicancy (p. 4). However, the detailed relief scheme it outlined aimed largely at managing beggars, and minimizing the social risks they appeared to pose. Birth control did not figure in the long-term suggestions that were presented to the Committee. Some accounts accepted the 'beggar problem' to be an outcome of the population pressure and consequent unemployment, but suggested agricultural modernization and employment generation as solutions (*ND* 18 February 1941: 2; 2 August 1941: 5; 2 September 1941: 2). Others linked such destitution with the impact of the war on the local economy, and the fall in prices for local products (*ND* 20 August 1941: 2). Practical efforts to manage the destitute were largely limited to help provided by relief committees, establishment of destitute homes, charity by various organizations, issue of begging permits, and the like.[6]

In each of these contexts, the rising population was unambiguously identified as one of the primary roots of the particular malaise under scrutiny. However, this did not mean that the merits of population management as a developmental measure became immediately evident. Even when this was conceded, it was inserted into a much larger plan of development almost inevitably, along with major interventions in agriculture and industry. Indeed, it could not be pushed as valuable in itself, but only as a measure bolstering a larger effort. As the communist member of the Travancore–Cochin Legislative Assembly, E. Gopalakrishna Menon, emphatically put it: 'when the government says that population must be controlled without any real basis or plan, I consider it to be an insult to the people of this country.' (*Proceedings of the Travancore–Cochin Legislative Assembly* 1952: 1601–2). Much of the pro-population control writing and speeches of the late 1950s and 1960s projected FP precisely in this way, as a useful tool, but certainly not capable of replacing industrialization or modernization of agriculture. Nevertheless, FP began to secure a special place in popular projections of the developmentalist agenda in subtle ways. First, it began to be persistently projected as a more 'fundamental' measure, to be implemented as a prior condition to the later interventions, as if the actualization of the latter depended on the success of the former. Innumerable articles, speeches, appeals, and exhortations that appeared in the Malayalam media in the late 1950s and 1960s elaborated this projection.[7] Secondly, it was projected as the cheapest, easiest, and most immediate 'contribution' that the individual could make. All that seemed to be required for such acceptance seemed the generation of a certain 'enlightened consciousness' and awareness of self-interest that would prompt the individual to take up this cause with zest (for instance, as argued by the family planning propagator, S. Krishna Kumar, in Kumar 1971). Thirdly, the machinery to channel this effort at popularization appeared particularly well developed in Malayali society. Its large network of civil organizations included not just upper- and upper-middle class associations like the Lions' and Rotary Clubs, Junior Chambers of Commerce, and the like, but also, and far more numerously, the local units of community-organizations and women's associations. Besides, the network of the institutions of modern health-care was also well developed and actively used (Jeffrey 2003: 192). While developmentalist intervention in agriculture or industry seemed more actively mediated by political society, FP appeared to be the one developmentalist activity that could be effectively mediated by civil society. Easily classifiable under 'health' or 'domestic well being', FP somehow seemed less prone to contention and politics.

These arguments became all the more persuasive under certain politico–economic conditions, which made industrialization, intensified agriculture, and other such recommendations appear rather difficult and, indeed, distant. This will be examined in detail in the following section.

Tiding Over Disenfranchisement

By the early 1960s, however, it was becoming amply clear that the vision of becoming enfranchised citizens of the Indian nation, so ardently cherished in the Malayali public sphere, was receding somewhat alarmingly. At the same time, the large population was not bringing any gains to the state. Several editorials, articles, and speeches from the early 1950s onwards had persistently claimed that Malayalis deserved greater allocations in the central budget, being more populous and 'backward' than other regions; these appeals seemed completely ineffectual. The sense of being a periphery both in a geographical and economic sense is acute in these texts. A sense of injustice in central allocations was further accentuated by pointing to Kerala's contribution to India's foreign exchange earnings. In the early years, this was often accompanied by the assertion of the 'superiority' of the Malayalis who, it was claimed, were more modernized than others. Responding to the Krishnamachari Committee's suggestions regarding financial merger, P. Balakrishnan, a member of the Travancore–Cochin State Legislative Assembly expressed his indignation: 'Do inform the members of that Committee and those who appointed them that we are not to be treated like the people of Northern India. Our culture is very different from the rustic culture of Northern India ... [they] must not be allowed to insult us thus, we, who deserve a prime position in culture and civilization ...' (*ND* 13 August 1949: 9). While this sense of superiority barely surfaces in the later years, the claim to be active contributors (as producers of foreign exchange-generating cash crops) was made ever more shrilly. In the mid-1960s, the anguished sense of isolation; of having to undertake the journey towards economic growth *alone*, was very prominant in Malayalam newspapers. The *Matrubhumi* protested angrily over the disappointing allocation to Kerala in the Fourth Plan, in an editorial entitled 'A Cruel Joke':

> The Advisory Committee had prepared a Plan of 1020 crores for Kerala ... but the National Planning Commission must have laughed seeing those figures! So much? For Kerala? If the resources earmarked for the Draft Fourth Plan are shared proportionate to population size, then Kerala would deserve somewhat that amount. But who cares for the population of Kerala? ... We will not say that Kerala is dependent on India the same way India is dependent on foreign nations. But seeing the tug-of-war between the states, and the helplessness of the Centre, we feel that we may have to largely rely upon ourselves. Our problems will not remain problems if each citizen of Kerala would act in his respective field with full honesty and to the best of his abilities. [17 November 1966: 6.]

Angry retorts to statements made about Kerala's 'problems' by functionaries of the union government implicitly referred to the superiority of the people of Kerala. Responding to the union planning minister Asoka Mehta's statement that all states claim to be short of resources, an author in *Matrubhumi* reminded its readers that '... Kerala is rich. Here, efficient and intelligent people are born. However, most of them are toiling in other lands to develop the wealth of those regions.... No remedy to this seems immediately in sight.' (13 November 1966: 11.) It is also striking that the political class in Kerala was frequently blamed for its inability to actively and shrewdly negotiate with the union authorities in the allocation of funds and location of industries.[8]

A second backdrop against which this sense of frustration and isolation grew was the severe food crisis. The shaping of the food crisis in India was itself intimately related to the developmental strategies chosen by the Indian nation-state and to the particular US- centred food regime that emerged in the post- Second World War decades (Frankel 1971; 1978, Gupta 1999). The drastic failure of the agricultural policies of the Second Five-Year Plan resulted in a fall in grain production by 10 per cent between 1956–7 and 1957–8. Food prices jumped by 50 per cent, the government had to import 6 million tons of food grains in two years, drawing on the PL 480 wheat. In the mid-1960s, it was clear that increases in agricultural output were not happening. The monsoon failed for two critical years, 1965–6 and 66–7, sharply bringing down the food grain output. This led to heavy imports, which rose from 3.1 million tons of wheat in 1956–7 to 10 million in 1965–6. The public distribution system became almost entirely dependent on PL 480 wheat. The war with Pakistan in 1965 led to the suspension of food aid by the US, and the politically-fraught decision to devalue the currency was made in June 1966 (Gupta 1999: 60).

These difficult national circumstances manifested all the more painfully in Kerala, which had been a food deficit state for very long, and dependent on imports. Public debate in Kerala on this issue in these years, again, brims with the deep sense of resentment against being relegated to beggar-status, notwithstanding Kerala's valuable contribution to India's foreign exchange resources. Even nationalist newspapers like *Matrubhumi* spouted ire in rhetoric that came quite close to being anti-Indian. Protesting the reduction of rice-rations to 4 ounces and wheat to 6 ounces for Kerala, it launched a veritable tirade:

> Such experiences ought to set Malayalis thinking. Our large population is a danger. Let it be so. Whether it was for ourselves or for others, it was certainly a major change when we began to grow cash crops in food croplands. The advantage from such crops depends on prices in the world market. We understand that even if the prices are high, money is not edible. Experts often come here to advise us that Kerala should not abandon profit-making, foreign-exchange-earning cash crops and concentrate on grains, and write

> reports [in that vein]. But why do they not come to teach us that groundnuts, tea, coffee or rubber can be eaten in the place of rice ... We are of course learning through our bitter experiences that unification and integration are all moving along one direction alone! ... we would have understood if this situation was created out of the scarcity of rice in India. This 'unification' that is being imposed even when there is rice available, this is horrendous. [7 January 1966: 4.]

This is not to hint that there was a strong anti-Indian sentiment in Kerala in the context of the food crisis on the same scale, or of the same kind, cutting across established political affiliations. Indeed not. The strident demands made by the chief minister of Kerala, E.M.S. Nambutiripad, elicited sharp criticism that it had undesirable separatist overtones (*Matrubhumi* 9 June 1967: 4; 8 August 1967; *MM* 19 June 1967: 2). Yet there can be little doubt that the food crisis heightened the sense of the vulnerability of the Malayali people, especially in a context in which cash crop cultivation seemed to be proceeding quite unabated, even if the food crop yields had increased.[9] Indeed, these very years saw the intensification of the FP propaganda, which incessantly and perhaps quite effectively, drove home the point that the food crisis was essentially a product of the rising population.[10]

As for industrialization too, the prospects seemed to be waning. Developmentalist thinking in pre-Independence Kerala had identified industrialization as crucial to development in an economy characterized by excessive pressure of population on land (Rammohan 1996). P.T. Chacko, speaking in the Indian Constituent Assembly in 1949 against the proposed taxation of industry in the states by the central government emphasized this in unequivocal terms:

> Compared to other parts of India, Travancore is thickly populated. There are but one or two countries in the world that has figures of population per square mile comparable to Travancore. The majority of the people of the country are farmers ... The population of Travancore is rising, but the hardworking people have no land to cultivate. Their sole succour is industrialization.... As far as the people in this area are concerned, industrialization is a life-and-death issue. [*ND* 13 September 1949: 1.]

In this context, great hopes were placed on the Nehruvian nation-state's aid. Indeed, rapid economic development through accelerated industrialization was directly identified as the principal means through which the Malayali people could overcome their relative 'lacks', such as, for instance, being relatively small in terms of population and command over resources. In the 1950s and '60s, bitter reprimands about the central government's neglect of Kerala's need for industry, and its reluctance to locate large public sector units here were heard.[11] These were, again, directly linked to Kerala's marginality within the Indian nation: its inability to press its demands effectively. Again, the 'civilized' way in which Malayalis were making their demands to the central government was frequently contrasted to the crudity of other states, and the central government was even warned that self-control should not be taken for weakness. *Malayala Manorama*, commenting on the agitation in Andhra for the fourth steel plant, and on T. Amrita Rao's pressure tactics, found reasons to praise the Malayali people:

> Comparing Andhra and Kerala, one feels proud of the people and the students of Kerala. There is much more industrial backwardness in Kerala compared to Andhra. In the past three Five Year Plans, Kerala has been ignored. Even then, neither the people nor the students here have resorted to violent demonstrations. This surely shows higher standards of rationality and prudence ... [*MM* 2 November 1966: 2.]

In a veritable philippic against the central government's unfulfilled assurances, *Matrubhumi* warned it that it should, in the least, desist from making such assurances and raising effete hopes. '*Keraleeeyar* [the people of Kerala] may lack many things, but to date no one has found them lacking in intelligence. Do not mock their intelligence, do not insult it.' (5 June 1970: 4.) In the context of such frustration, the relevance of population control appeared doubled, in that it seemed a way of lowering the pressure of population on land, and upon the resources of the government, which could be diverted to industrialization. Precisely this was highlighted in E.M.S. Nambutiripad's speech in support of FP, broadcast during a FP Week celebration in 1967 (*Matrubhumi* 21 September 1967: 3).

Fourthly, the prospects of migration also seemed to be declining grievously. Earlier there was optimism that the problem of high population density could be resolved through migration towards other parts of India. *Prabhatam* tried to allay fears expressed in the Census Report of Cochin in 1945 by pointing out that '... some experts opine that given India's vastness and the prospects of migration to other areas within it, no one needs to be scared of rising population, and therefore the fears of the advocates of population control are baseless' (22 April 1945: 7). Internal migration had taken place in massive numbers to the hill areas within Travancore, Cochin, and Malabar, and to the adjacent areas such as Gudalloor, South Canara, and Shimoga in these decades. In the press as well as in the legislative bodies, the demand that the migration of Malayalis to other parts of India should be facilitated through government intervention was heard very frequently in the 1950s and early 1960s.[12] However, even the internal migrants, even those who had been encouraged to settle in the hill areas as cultivators by the government found themselves facing serious threat of eviction in the wake of food-production efforts of the 1940s, such as the Grow More Food Campaign. Settlers in the South Canara region, many of whom had established themselves there as part of the Madras government's food production efforts in the late 1940s, were facing the threat of eviction in the early 1960s.[13] Stories and editorials continued to appear in the Malayalam press through the 1960s right into the 1970s, for example, of the difficulties faced by Malayali farmer–emigrants, and the threats of eviction they faced in Shimoga, Gudalloor and in forest areas within Kerala.[14] However, migration continued to be advocated as an essential measure, a responsibility of the government, and one to be undertaken on a large scale. Thus in 1963, *Malayala Manorama* was recommending that the government must implement a planned migration programme in which 25 lakh Malayalis were to be resettled in thinly populated regions (editorial 30 January 1963: 2). Yet, by these years, it was becoming increasingly evident that the ideal powerful nation-state that would forcefully mediate the migration, and weld all the diversity and conflicting interests into national unity, was not a reality. Regional sentiments and centres of authority were posing almost insurmountable problems for easy migration. *Matrubhumi* reminded the authorities in 1969 about the Gudalloor evictions:

> Everyone knows the stories of the adventurous [people], who move away from thickly populated Kerala with the hunger for land, and go anywhere they can, clearing forests, leveling mountains, braving malaria and the inclemency of Nature to raise the flag of labour ... Until the state of Kerala was formed, Malabar and its other parts, as was Gudalloor Taluk, was part of the Madras Presidency. In that sense, those farmers who have laboured for many decades in the Nilgiri forests where death lies in wait, to create first-rate farmland to raise coffee, tea, coconut, arecanut and paddy were migrating within their own State. If they have come to become aliens in their own soil now, they should surely be not faulted for it. [*Matrubhumi* 19 September 1969: 4.]

Not surprisingly, *Kerala Kaumudi* compared the move to evict 5000 families from Gudalloor with the efforts of the Siva Sena to displace south Indians in Mumbai (*KK* 10 September 1971: 2). These were also times in which the weakness of the Indian nation-state's inability to contain the upsurge of regional sentiments was beginning to show. These tensions were often directed against people of other regions, as in the attacks on south Indians in Mumbai in 1969, which drew considerable ire in the Malayalam press.[15] Anger against the central government in the press was scarcely concealed on this issue:

> Malayalis have suffered tremendous losses in this riot.... The number of Malayalis trying to return to Kerala is not negligible. As far as Kerala is concerned this is a life-and-death issue. As far as Malayalis are Indian citizens they must [have] the facility and the right to live and work in any part of this country. This right has to be assured by the government of India. If the government cannot assure that, then Malayalis are not obliged to pay taxes, reckoning this government to be theirs, or live in the illusion that this great country is their mother land. The central government must realize that Malayalis have extremely intense emotions in this issue. [*KK* 20 February 1969: 2.]

Besides this, it appeared that even in the 'colonization' programmes undertaken by the central government, Kerala was being given a raw deal, notwithstanding its claims to being the most thickly populated region. In the Dandakaranya Programme, refugees from East Pakistan were apparently given precedence, and only a relatively minor share was allotted to Kerala (*MM* 10 December 1960: 6). It was claimed that Malayalis, who were efficient farmers, and seeking land, were being sidelined in favour of refugees from East Pakistan, who either did not want to migrate at all, or were being prevented somehow from doing so (*MM* 18 September 1964: 2). By the end of the 1960s, the state government was conceding its helplessness in this regard. In response to a question in the State Legislative Assembly, minister M.K. Krishnan replied that the distribution of land in the Andaman Islands was contingent upon the decisions of the central government. He clarified that the central government was apparently planning to settle refugees from Burma there, and that it was fruitless for the state government to prepare such programmes by itself (*Proceedings of the Kerala State Legislative Assembly* 1967: 3487–8). The prominent Congress leader from Kerala, C.M. Stephen, even declared in parliament in despair that Malayalis were refugees within their own country, who, received much less attention than refugees from East Bengal (*Matrubhumi* 9 June 1971: 1).

Thus, by the 1960s, all the developmental measures that had been proposed earlier as possible solutions to the problem of high population density seemed to be either far too distant or moving at a decidedly tepid pace. The desirability of FP seemed utterly self-evident in this context. The advocacy of FP was characterized by an unmistakable ambivalence. On the one hand, much of the FP propaganda called upon 'enlightened' and 'educated' Malayali to embrace family regulation, as if only such assent would operate as irrefutable proof of the presence of such superior qualities as the above, among the Malayalis. In many such accounts, there appears to be virtually a seamless continuity between the development-conscious Malayali, and the responsible Indian citizen, the interests of one complementing the other. The alleged reluctance of

Malayalis to adopt FP as a developmental instrument worked in such accounts to exonerate the government(s) from blame regarding the lack of development, and this argument was employed even by caustic critics of the inertia of government(s) such as *Matrubhumi*. At the eve of the 1967 elections, one of its editorials drew upon the high-population thesis to exculpate the Congress government at the centre of the developmental failures in Kerala. It claimed that India's situation has not improved significantly in the past eighteen years, and held the increase in population squarely responsible for this. The government had magnanimously refrained from coercion, yet the people did not enthusiastically welcome its population management initiatives. Catholics and the Muslim League were singled out for blame, for not offering immediate and direct support. 'The national income has gone up by 69 per cent. If it has not increased more, it is because we have overbred. It is not the government, which has provided ample facilities for Family Planning that is to be blamed, but ourselves.' (Editorial, 14 February 1967: 3.) After the successful mass sterilization camp at Ernakulam in 1971, the Health Minister of Kerala, N.K. Balakrishnan, jubilantly translated the 'births averted' into material terms, again, assuming uninterrupted continuity between the interests of the Indian nation-state and the Malayalis, and also a smooth flow of resources from the Centre to the state:

> According to the Indian government's figures, three births are averted through one sterilization surgery. It is calculated that the government spends Rs 3500 per child through government budgets until it attains 20 years of age (besides the sum the parents spend). Over 2 lakh births have been averted through the approximately 80,000 sterilization surgeries performed in the two Camps. By this the government has gained 75 crores. That is, the cost of building two ship-building yards have been gained. [*Matrubhumi* 2 August 1971: 2.]

With this, the status of FP as an instrument for development became established as an almost unassailable truth. A legislator in the Legislative Assembly of Kerala even asseverated that the victorious mass sterilization camps at Ernakulam represented 'an achievement greater than what would be attained through a Five-

Year Plan', and prominent sections of the media agreed with him (*Matrubhumi* 22 July 1971: 2). Notwithstanding the general commitment to avoidance of coercion, recommendations of compulsory sterilisation and other coercive measures were not unheard of.[16]

On the other hand, the espousal of FP was often clearly admitted to be part of a survival strategy in the face of an extremely adverse situation, part of which at least was a direct outcome of the marginal position of Malayalis within the Indian nation. It was plainly acknowledged that neither agriculture nor industry was really taking off in Kerala, nor were opportunities for migration broadened. In these accounts, FP appears to be a measure grasped in desperation to reach the goal of development against all odds; to emerge victorious in a lone battle waged by the Malayalis in which they had no dependable allies. Such an admission regarding the crisis of development in Kerala, as quoted below, was by no means an exception:

> Though the major occupation of the people is agriculture, a situation of land scarcity has been prevailing here from earlier on. Neither have we been able to increase job opportunities through industrialization. Because of this, food scarcity and unemployment have become incurable ailments. [*Kerala Kaumudi* 12 July 1971: 2.]

However, the malady of rising numbers is immediately seized upon as the root cause of the crisis, and the fundamental groundbreaking solution is identified to lie in popularization of FP. The editorial continues: 'The root of all our present-day sufferings is the increase in population. If we are able to implement the FPP effectively, then the solutions to other problems will work out by themselves' (p. 2). The necessity of FP is sometimes presented as one of the lessons learned from the bitter experience of 'national integration', which seemed not so much to enfranchise Malayalis as able citizens of the developing nation, as to disenfranchise them. The failure of the nation-state to create a 'neutral space' of development, which those who had to cut loose from their regional moorings could safely inhabit, was recognized as a reality, and reducing numbers was hailed as a wise response.

So also was the painful realization that the Nehruvian possibility of the national community that was to be brought into being through uniform development, in which the more-developed regions would pitch in and help their poorer neighbours, was ebbing away. In these contexts, it seemed necessary to turn 'inward' to find the energy and the resources for development. The promotion of FP was an integral part of this manoeuvre. As *Kerala Kaumudi* remarked:

> It is fruitless to say that India is one and that we are citizens of this vast India. Malayalis, Tamilians and Maharashtrians … are Indian citizens. In the struggle to survive, no one will make a concession to anyone else. Each one will have to look after his own interests. Malayalis must seek to remedy their unemployment by themselves. Moreover, that should be within Kerala itself. In order to be invited to the feast, there must be sufficient food in the house. Our immediate duty is to prevent the rise of population in Kerala and to implement agricultural and industrial programmes that will increase employment opportunities. [*Kerala Kaumudi* 20 July 1969: 2.]

In this section, the effort has been to sketch the larger politico–economic context in which the (sub-)nationality of Kerala took shape, which was important in making FP appear as an essential component of the economic solution to Kerala's growth-indisposition. The specific context sketched out above had a critical role to play in projecting FP as a viable and desirable economic solution. This, no doubt, was only a conspicuous element in a entire 'bundle' of strategies of (re)presentation. FP was at times tied to the aspiration of 'responsible parenting', which had been gaining circulation quite steadily in Malayali society from the early decades of the twentieth century onwards. It was at times tied to depoliticized notions of 'uplift', 'self-help', and even to a circumscribed 'liberation', accessing the missionary-mode of drawing subjects, which was already quite familiar to Malayalis for almost a century. However, the successful promotion of the FPP was also related to the politico–economic predicament that was widely believed to exist in especially intensified proportions in the 1960s, which made a case for viewing birth control as an important developmental intervention.[17]

This makes the FPP an important event in the history of developmentalism in Malayali society too. It is of course is distinct from the view that the successful FPP in Kerala produced important economic spin-offs that would fructify later. Developmentalism was crucial to the shaping of the modern Malayali identity; the preservation of the developmentalist aspiration through the FPP was important in shaping the specific ideological responses within Malayali political society to the decline of the Nehruvian vision of the developmentalist nation-state. I would also argue that the FPP was a revealing moment in the history of civil social activism in Kerala. More of this however in the next and concluding section.

Preserving Developmentalism

By the mid-1960s, it was very evident that the Nehruvian vision of the developmentalist nation was declining. The Chinese war marked the disillusionment with the Nehruvian era of rule; drought, economic strain, and war forced a break in planned development. Now, the idealized project of 'national development' had to negotiate with various localized claims to local resources, which manifested in movements that aggressively projected regional identities, and directed this against people of other regions. Moreover, the Nehruvian vision of balanced economic growth throughout the subcontinent with large-scale public sector industrialization and the nation-state playing a commanding role seemed to be fading. War, drought, and subsequent food crises brought into full view the plight of peripheral, food-deficient, non-industrialized areas like Kerala. This period also saw the re-legitimation of the jingoistic Hindu right and its vision of the nation as *punyabhoo* (holy land), especially in the northern heartland and in the western parts of India.

The terrible anxieties over development expressed in the Malayali public sphere of the 1960s may be read in this context. Considering the degree to which the energetic articulation of a modern Malayali identity had been tied to vigorous and egalitarian economic development of Kerala, the highly tenebrous mood in the Malayalam press is almost predictable. On the one hand, the dream of realizing an egalitarian community of patriotic producers, whose Malayali identity would by no means clash with citizenship in the developing nation, seemed increasingly implausible. On the other hand, the prospect of building an economically self-sufficient regional political unit above threats from its (better-endowed) neighbours seemed bleaker than ever. Almost the entire spectrum of forces inhabiting Malayali political society seemed discredited. First, they had failed in securing the economic interests of Kerala in their negotiations with the nation-state. Secondly, they were held responsible for releasing a host of 'political problems', ranging from squabbles over sharing the government, thereby preventing the establishment of stable government, to political interference in developmental initiatives, to fostering a certain 'overpoliticization' which was seen to be hampering the economic development of the state.

At this particularly difficult juncture in the history of egalitarian developmentalism in the late 1960s–early '70s in Kerala, the FPP and the land reforms proved momentous. The FPP appeared to be offering the means to tide over both anxieties. On the one hand, it kept alive, as an ideology, the promise of development, continuing to offer the prospect of mobilizing resources from within, a point that was incessantly hammered in as part of the FPP propaganda. On the other hand, it united political society, to a considerable degree. Large sections of political society had already quite vocally declared their allegiance to the FPP. Though the active presence of dissenting voices was indeed important in keeping the FPP less coercive than elsewhere, concerted opposition from within political society was much weaker here. If the promise of development was sheltered by the FPP campaign, the promise of egalitarian ideology was kept burning by the land reforms, and this actualized through political society and under its scrutiny. This is not to claim that the FPP campaign and the land reforms were deliberately deployed as strategies to prop up such ideologies; only that this was not the least negligible among their effects.

After the 1970s, egalitarian developmentalism, which had been the common rallying point for civil, social, and political institutions here, began to be questioned more frequently, and from different perspectives. In such critical evaluations, the ineffectiveness of political society in delivering its promises, as well as the unrealistic and environmentally improvident developmental ambitions it fostered, became the target of new critiques from civil society.[18] However, the forceful interventions of civil social actors into the discourse of development did not unseat certain dominant features of developmentalism in any significant sense: as, for instance, its adherence to gender roles. For instance, the 'People's Science Movement', the Kerala Sastra Sahitya Parishat, operated within the terms of developmentalism even as it powerfully questioned the dominance of political society, articulating alternative visions and means. Thus it is no surprise that a major study on the KSSP preferred to refer to it as a 'development movement' (Zacharia and Sooryamurthy 1994). I argue that the success of the FPP and the land reforms were crucial in preserving the fortunes of egalitarian developmentalism as the reigning ideology of the élites in Kerala. The élitism and gender blindness of devlopmentalism continued to inform the discourse of 'social development', and later the discourse of 'human development' centred upon Kerala's experience of development. Also, civil social activism (not just by élite circles like the Lions' or Rotary Clubs, but also by radical intellectuals and non-élite, rural groups and associations) was mobilized to developmentalist ends in an unprecedented way during the FPP. This was to have a crucial impact on the shape that civil social interventions in developmentalist discourse and practice was to take in Kerala in the later decades. Thus the FPP remains a crucial event in the histories of developmentalism and civil social mobilizations in Kerala in the latter half of the twentieth century, often serving to highlight the interconnections of the two. Being so closely integrated with the developmentalist project, civil social movements in Kerala did not really unseat the widespread abhorrence of those aspects of modernity that seemed conducive to individual autonomy, especially that of women. This is of crucial importance when we consider the way in which artificial contraception continues to be translated solely as 'family planning' in Kerala. Loosening patriarchal control over reproduction has never figured very high in the agendas of these movements.

To say this, then, is to indicate that the politico–social impact of the successful FPP in Kerala exceeds the economic benefits or ills that may have resulted from the quickening of demographic transition. This, of course, is an issue for further and sustained historical research effort, which may well reveal surprising and counter-intuitive connections in the historical shaping of Kerala's present.

Notes

[1] I use the term '(sub-)national' to indicate that the appeals to patriotic Malayalis were not really directed *against* the Indian nation-state, in the sense of proposing secession, though they were undoubtedly critical of the central government's neglect of Kerala's development.

[2] See, for instance, report of speech in the Sree Mulam Praja Sabha by Vettikkattu Antony Varghese, *Nazrani Deepika* (henceforth, *ND*) 9 April 1929: 6; editorial, *ND*, 14 February 1936, 2; K.S. Nair, 'Anchukaranangal Grammenadhapatanattinu' (Five reasons for the decline of villages), *ND*,17 July 1941, 3; P.R. Sankarappillai, 'Shreevazhumkotile Gramajeevitam' (Rural life in Travancore), 10 November 1941 *ND*: 2; August 1953, 4.

[3] Changanashery Parameshwaran Pillai, 'Janavardhana' (Increase in population), *Kutumbapatrika* 2,7, 1934, 8, recommended migration; such suggestions became far more numerous in the 1950s. See, for a few instances, *ND* 24 June 1952, 2; 'F.C', *ND* 30 September 1954, 2; report of speech by Union Planning Minister G.L. Nanda, *ND* 3 November 1954, 1; report of speeches at the Nair Conference at Tiruvalla, *ND* 17 May 1955, 2; V.V. Giri, press statement, *Malayalarajyam* 4 July 1961, 2. Intensive agriculture was too frequently recommended to be cited; however, a few instances may be mentioned: *ND* 23 September 1926, 6; Dr P.J. Thomas, speech at the Ernakulam Village Uplift Conference, *ND* 1 February 1939, 2; K.E. Job, Dr Kurialasery Memorial Lecture, *ND* 2 August 1941, 4; speech by the Finance Secretary, *ND* 22 July 1941, 3; E. M. S. Nambutiripad, 'Kazhinja 30 Varsham Chatuppu- Innu Punchiritookum Pacchappadam' (Swamp since the last 30 Years—now a green field beaming bright) [1944], in P.Govinda Pillai (ed.) *E.M.S. Sampoorna Kritikal 1952–53* Vol. XIII, Thiruvananthapuram, Chinta, 2000, 83–6; I.C. Chacko, 'Krishivikasanam; Pambapaddhatikalum Mattu Paddhatikalum'(Agricultural development: the Pampa and other projects), *ND* 11 May 1949, 1; editorial, *Malayala Manorama* 19 March 1960: 2; editorial, *Matrubhumi*, 30 December 1965, 4.

[4] J.C. Kumarappa, speech, *Matrubhumi* 4 June 1950, 6; M.P. Manmadhan, speech, *Malayala Manorama* (henceforth, *MM*) 25 April 1969, 4; E. Ikkanda Warrier, speech, *Matrubhumi*, 26 March 1962, 4.

[5] P.K. Sukumaran, 'Santananiyantranamo Sambattikasootranamo?' (Birth control or economic planning?), *Janayugam* Onam Special Number, 1963, 115–17; P.J. Thomas, discussion on the food deficit organized by the University Research

Organisation at Thiruvananthapuram, *ND* 29 September 1951: 2; speech at the Workers' School at Thrissur, *ND* 6 June 1950: 1; also see, Puttezhattu Raman Menon, 'Janapperuppavum Bhakshanakshamavum' (Population increase and food shortage), in *Arivulla Ajnanikal*, Kottayam, SPSS, [1955] 1970, 72-92; also his 'Onam!!' and 'Kritrima Ari' (Artificial rice) in *Parihasattiloote*, Kottayam, SPSS, 1969, 1–29, 228–38.

6 See, *ND* 1 October 1941, 3; 19 May 1941, 6, on the issue of begging permits; report on Beggar Relief Home at Kottayam, *ND* 3 January 1941, 1; discussion on the resolution on Beggar Relief Centres, K.R. Narayanan, 30 August 1944, *Proceedings of the Travancore Sree Mulam Assembly* Vol. XX, 1945, 976–98; discussion of the Travancore Prevention of Begging Bill brought by N. Ramakrishna Pillai, 20 February 1945, *Proceedings of the Travancore Sree Mulam Assembly* Vol. XXV, 1946, 166–71; report on charity work at Chertala by the members of the Maramon parish, *ND* 12 February 1941, 3, on the relief committee established by the Travancore State Congress to prevent starvation at Cherthala.

7 See, for instance, Kuttippuzha Krishna Pillai, 'Jananniyantranam' (1962), in *Kuttippuzhayute Prabandhangal* Vol III (Essays of Kuttippuzha), Thrissur, Kerala Sahitya Akademi, 1990, 121–5; editorial, *Malayala Rajyam* 26 August 1964, 1; K.R. Narayanan, 'Janasankhya Ingane Perukiyal!' (If population grows like this!), *MM* Sunday Supplement, 14 August 1966, I; editorial, *Kerala Kaumudi* 5 Aug. 1967, 2; editorial, *Kerala Kaumudi* 15 February 1968, 2; K. Peetambaran, *Kutumbasootranam* (Family Planning), Kottayam, SPSS, 1969; editorial, *Kerala Kaumudi* 13 December 1969, 2; editorial, *Matrubhumi* 7 December 1969, 4; 'Ernakulatte Kootavasectomy' (Mass sterilization at Ernakulam), *Matrubhumi* 26 July 1971, 3; editorial, *Kerala Kaumudi* 28 October 1971, 2.

8 See, for a few instances, editorial, *ND* 19 July 1954, 2; editorial, *MM* 20 November 1958, 2; *ND* 22 September 1960, 3; *Kerala Kaumudi*, 7 September 1961, 2; editorial, *Matrubhumi* 31 July 1966, 4; editorial, *Matrubhumi* 7 September 1966, 6; editorial, *MM* 2 July 1969, 4; 9 January 1967, 2; editorial, *Matrubhumi* 7 May 1970, 3; editorial, *Kerala Kaumudi* 28 December 1967, 2.

9 There was considerable euphoria about the success of the high-yielding variety of rice (see, editorial, *MM* 6 May 1966, 2), but also equal misgivings about the actual benefits to be reaped from it. However, the fear that it was not at all suited to the region, and that people were not prepared to buy the rice, was widely expressed (editorial, *MM* 19 June 1967, 2). There was also scepticism about the benefits of improved rice yields at the national level for Kerala. See, editorial, *Kerala Kaumudi* 13 August 1968, 2.

10 See, for instance, editorial, *Kerala Kaumudi* 15 February 1968, 2; speech by advisor to Kerala, N.E.S. Raghavachari, *Matrubhumi*, 12 December 1966, 5; editorial, *Matrubhumi* 29 July 1968, 4; K.R. Narayanan, 'Janasankya Ingane Perukiyal!' (If population grows thus!), *MM*, Sunday Supplement, 14 August 1966, 1; speech by secretary of the Health Department, C.K. Kochukoshy,

MM, Sunday Supplement, 18 September 1966, 1.

[11] See, *ND* 26 June 1954, 3–6; editorial, *MM* 20 November 1958, 2; editorial, *MM* 15 January 1959, 2; M.A. Oommen, 'Dhanakaryacommissionum Keralavum' (The Finance Commission and Kerala), *MM* Sunday Supplement 8 October 1961, I; editorial, *MM* 28 July 1961, 2; editorial, *MM* 18 October 1961, 2; report of protest by members of parliament from Kerala, *MM* 6 October 1964, 2; editorial, *Kerala Kaumudi* 13 January 1967, 2; editorial, *Matrubhumi* 7 May 1970, 3.

[12] See, report of prospects of migration to Borneo, *ND* 22 July 1952, 5; 'Andamans Kutiyetta Paddhati' (Plan for migration to the Andamans) *ND* 13 May 1953, 1; editorial *ND* 23 January 1955, 2; P.J. Thomas, article on prospects of migration to Brazil as farmers, *ND* 11 November 1958, 2; 'Dandakaranya Paddhatiyum Keralavum' (Kerala and the Dandakaranya Project), *MM* 17 November 1960, 6; editorial, *ND* 14 September 1960, 2; report of question and answer in Kerala State Legislative Assembly, *MM* 21 December 1961, 2; speech by Governor V.V. Giri, *MM* 2 July 1961, 1; editorial, *MM* 1 May 1962, 2; V.V.Giri, speech, *MM*, 31 January 1963, 1; reply to starred question no. 1247 on colonization in the Kerala State Legislative Assembly, 1 August 1967, *Proceedings of the Kerala Legislative Assembly* Vol. XXI, 1968, 3487–88; editorial, *Matrubhumi* 27 July 1969, 4.

[13] Reported in the *MM* 9 October 1960, 1; editorial, *ND* 8 October 1960, 2; editorial, *MM* 11 October 1960, 4.

[14] See for instance, appeal by Marayur Karshaka Sanghom, *ND* 6 April 1957, 2; memorandum from the Kandallur Colony Karshaka Samajam, *ND* 12 March 1958, 2; article on forest encroachment in the High Ranges, *MM* 7 May 1960, 2; editorial, *MM* 15 January 1963, 2; editorial, *MM* 27 April 1963, 2; report from Kallarkutty, *MM* 13 December 1963, 4; *MM* 5 May 1966, 2; *Matrubhumi* 26 February 1966, 2; editorial, *Matrubhumi* 19 September 1969,4; *Kerala Kaumudi* 10 September 1971, 2.

[15] See, editorial, *Kerala Kaumudi* 13 August 1967, 2; editorial, *Kerala Kaumudi*, 25 May 1968, 2, article, 'Malayalikal Marumnattil' (Malayalis abroad), *Kerala Kaumudi* 26 September 1968, 2. Besides the limited resettlement of a few Malayali families in Bhopal in the 1950s did not appear very successful now. See, report, *MM* 17 May 1966, 3.

[16] Report of the recommendations of the State-level FP Seminar at Thiruvananthapuram, *Matrubhumi* 14 January 1966, 4; Dr C.O. Karunakaran, 'Kutumbasootrana Paddhati' (The FPP), *Kerala Kaumudi* 11 March 1967, 2; 'Kutumbasootrananttinte Pracharanam' (Propagating FP), *Matrubhumi*, 15 July 1965, 5; A.P. Jain, governor of Kerala, speech endorsing government decision to deny maternity benefits to employees beyond the third pregnancy at FP Seminar at Thiruvananthapuram, reported in *Matrubhumi*, 24 December 1965, 1; Pamban Madhavan, statement in the Kerala Legislative Assembly, in favour of compulsory sterilization; O. Koran, statement, Kerala Legislative Assembly, favouring child-

tax, both in *Matrubhumi* 1 March 1962, 6; Dr M. K. Muhammad Sahir, speech at FP Camp at Thrissur favouring child-tax, *Malayala Rajyam* 28 March 1963, 4; speech by high court judge K. Sadasivan, *Matrubhumi* 30 September 1967, 6.

[17] There were, however, rare voices, not of well-known opponents of artificial contraception, like the Catholic Church, which were uneasy about the 'negativity' they perceived in the projection of birth control as a developmental strategy for overcoming the problem of overpopulation. For instance, the radical intellectual M. Gangadharan, writing in 1974 about what he perceived to be 'the greatest crisis Malayalis had ever faced', remarked that 'A tendency to behave defensively even in the face of this threat is taking shape here. The increasing inclination towards sterilization and abortions indicates this. But it does not seem possible to find a solution to the problem of overpopulation through merely a defensive response.' M. Gangadharan, 'Keraleeyata' [1974], in *Anveshanam, Asvadanam*, Kottayam, SPSS, 1980, 44.

[18] The struggle against the large-scale hydroelectric project proposed at Silent Valley in the early 1980s brought about a sharp polarization between the two visions of development, and civil social opponents of the Nehruvian vision of economic development won a major victory.

Conclusion

Pulling Together the Threads

To argue that such processes as those discussed in the preceding chapters have been crucial to the success of the FPP in the 1960s and early 1970s is to place it within the emergent material, and also the political, and ideological scenario of mid-twentieth century Malayali society. This is distinct from the familiar practice of explaining the success by culling out certain social features that hasten fertility decline, leaving the matrices of power within which it was shaped relatively untouched. For instance, it is certainly true to say that high female literacy made possible the acceptance of FP. Nevertheless, to stop there would be to ignore the wider politico–economic conditions, the new ways of viewing the self, the new forms of hierarchy, and the transformation of the domestic space within which FP came to be perceived as not only desirable, but also necessary. The dominant wisdom on FP in Malayali society shares the political blindness that was the hallmark of the FPP propaganda. Indeed, when politics is addressed, the tendency to rely upon a narrative of freedom-from-traditional bondage is apparent even in recent work (for instance, Leiten 2002). Here I have argued that the garnering of public consent for FPP was poised upon extensive changes in a number of crucial notions and institutions that cannot be encapsulated within such a simplistic frame of reference. The use of such a narrative as a Procrustean bed, which generates historical explanation by either convenient stretching or lopping, is challenged here. For instance, the early misgivings about artificial contraception are not accurately described as a fear of modernity: such fear was certainly more complicated. Rather, it was the anxiety that some elements of modernity might thwart a full-fledged developmental modernity that is found expressed in the publicly-expressed misgivings about artificial birth control and state support for it.

In the dominant view, the ambiguities of 'liberation' are entirely sidelined. First, tied as it was to the interests of productivist nation-building, the FPP propaganda remained largely uninterested in the expansion of individual choice in any effective sense; the 'liberation' from tradition meant not the end of constraint but insertion into the disciplinary regime of the productivist nation. The widespread availability of artificial contraception did not mean the substantial expansion of women's access to these. They were limited to married women, and the massive rise in female sterilizations since the late 1970s, which continues to this day, is also revealing. This does not however mean that women were always mere passive recipients, victims of a medicalizing juggernaut. Indeed, there are indications that further investigation into oral sources may unearth an almost wholly untold story of how women tried to fight off one kind of patriarchal institution (usually the closer one, that of the family/community) using others (the medical establishment and the state). A gynaecologist who was actively involved in the IUD insertion drives of the late 1960s in Kerala revealed that FP workers of the period often actively supported women's attempts to subvert their husbands' and in-laws' control over their fertility. This doctor herself mentioned several instances of women running into the FP clinic and requesting the attendants there to quickly insert the IUD, saying that they had come without the permission of the husband and in-laws. If the insertion was done at once, they pleaded, it would be possible to return home in time and avoid suspicion.[1] As feminist researchers in fertility studies have remarked, newer contraceptive technologies were easier to conceal, and women often used them to gain control of their fertility, keeping it concealed from husbands or in-laws (Bledsoe et al. 1994; Kaler 2000). However, there were other doctors who did not encourage such collusion, as was indicated in the first chapter.

Secondly, it may be true, as a prominent scholar has argued, that the labouring poor began to avail of artificial contraception when it seemed as though '... ascribed characters are subordinate to acquired ones so it helped them to be less fatalistic, and induced them to make an important switch from the quantity to the quality of children' (K.C. Zachariah, quoted in Bhat and Rajan 1990: 35). However, the acceptance of FP by the poor was certainly not a result of the spread of a radical consciousness sprung out of a lightening of life's burdens for the non-élites; of the ability to critically engage with institutions, old or new, among them. It was into the dominant culture of the educated middle-classes, characterized by modern patriarchy, developmentalism, and the élitism of modern knowledge that the labouring poor were 'liberated'. Indeed, the hypothesis that the widespread acceptance of FP by the poorest in Kerala was poverty-driven seems plausible in a certain sense,[2] but perhaps we ought to say insecurity-driven rather than poverty-driven. Militant struggles of the 1950s and 1960s culminated in the 1970s in the land reforms and the Agricultural Wage Workers Act, which gave legal status as 'permanent worker', along with a guaranteed right to employment to any worker who had worked on a particular landowner's property by custom, contract, or otherwise (Heller 1999: 138–9). However, the subsequent years saw the gradual erosion of permanency of work, which apparently got 'traded for wage increases' (Heller 1999: 145). In circumstances in which employment within agriculture did not rise, the workers were confronted with intense insecurities, even when they commanded higher wages. That of course is not to speak of the wider socio–cultural context in which manual work, however highly-paid, was increasingly stigmatized.

Besides, it is not as if 'becoming less fatalistic' and 'having new aspirations' happened outside the emergent ideological and social webs of power. It is not only that the coming of new personal aspirations entailed new responsibilities and anxieties, harder to recognize and resist, precisely because pleasure is harnessed to their fulfilment. That the space of the familial/personal, emergent in the struggles against the traditional order(s), heavily laden with the rhetoric of 'freedom', is conceived as one readily accessible to the modern state, is also important. The responsibility towards one's offspring was also tightly linked to responsibility to the state. I have argued that throughout the late nineteenth and twentieth centuries, in and through the process I have called 'domestication', the modern family has been configured as a matrix for organizing and coordinating domestic and conjugal arrangements not only in the name of the personal well-being of the individual members but also in the name of public citizenship (Rose 1996). In Malayali society in the course of the past century, we have seen sustained efforts to fuse the sense of the 'personal' to that of the 'familial' in an extraordinarily durable way. It is thus no surprise that we have come to perceive contraception as family planning, and to allow a convenience for family maintenance to stand in the place of an instrument of individual freedom.

Thus a dominant thread that runs through the chapters hints at the rooting of modern political rationality in which the object and target of governmental action is in some sense the necessary partner or accomplice of government. The process of 'domestication' is found central to this rooting. By the process of 'domestication', I mean a complex conjunction of discursive and non-discursive changes through which the major proportion of the energies, interests, desires, and commitments of individuals have been directed towards their immediate families, rather than the public. That this implies a solidification of modern gender may be evident. To be 'domesticated' was to be integrated into the modern domestic domain as responsible father/householder or mother/homemaker, engaged primarily in shaping children into productive (gendered) individuals.[3] Artificial contraception thus became a valued tool to this end. Indeed, the fear of 'loss of masculinity' in sterilization, while recorded in Kerala too (for instance, den Uyl 1995: 181) did not seem to affect the levels of male acceptance of vasectomy until after the National Emergency of 1975.[4] While this and other issues need to be investigated in much greater detail, one may well hypothesize that sterilization might not have evoked intense castration anxieties in the modern-educated Malayali male, at least in the 1960s. After all, the newer notions of masculinity were inextricably bound to the ability to support one's dependants within the nuclear family by one's self-earned income. This foregrounding of domestic concerns and obligations was carried forward actively in the 1970s through state-sponsored programmes like the mass sterilization camps, the One Lakh-Housing Scheme for the poor, and the Maveli stores, all which aimed at the consumption-oriented modernized (but poor) *family*.[5] Besides the hardening of the power-effects of modern gender relations, 'domestication' probably affected mobilization on behalf of larger collectivities such as the local community.

The question of resistance to governmental power has arisen in these chapters time and again without being directly addressed. Resistance was noted in the studies of the Demographic Research Centre; it, however, was conceived as something to be overcome through persuasion. Thus a 1969 study of knowledge and practice of FP in rural Kerala remarked thus: 'A large percentage of those who know the methods, do not practice them. Thus there is a wide gap between knowledge and practice of FP methods among the married couples in the rural areas. As the reason for non-practice of methods is not included in the enquiry it is not known why a large percentage refrain from practice in spite of their knowledge' (Nair and Nair 1978: 197).

Richer indications of resistance are however certainly present in the public discourse on FP. It surfaced, for instance, in some events that followed the successful Ernakulam mass sterilization camp of 1971, such as the formation of a 'union' of the sterilized, which demanded that the state compensate them for their 'sacrifices' for the nation. To mention another instance, in 1968, a frustrated FP worker wrote:

> During festivals like Onam, Christmas and other special occasions, women commonly approach FP centers more frequently to insert and remove IUDs. This is because they get paid for insertion. They claim an incentive from one FP center and get a loop inserted. When in need of money again, they

> put up false complaints like stomach pain and bleeding to get it removed. Then they go to another FP center, get an IUD inserted, claiming an incentive … [Letter to the Editor, *Matrubhumi* 18 January 1968: 4.]

Another point that I would argue for in the light of this enquiry relates to the importance of regarding the success of the FPP as an event of significance in the history of politics in Kerala. This should add an interesting spin to our investigations into the intersections of the historical trajectories of politics and development in Kerala. It is usually remarked that political differences hardly affected the pursuit of social development by rival governments in Kerala. The point raised here, however, goes on to claim that the FPP was a political event, in that it highlighted the centre–periphery relations in post-colonial India, the configurations of the individual, community, and state in mid-twentieth century Kerala, and informed the dynamics of civil and political societies in the decades to come. Thus there is need to qualify the current view that places it within the history of development in Kerala, in a way that assumes that it has little to do with politics.

Further Reflections

What other reflections emerge, then, from this historical exploration? What kinds of writing-work lie ahead of this effort that would extend and strengthen the critical effort? What are the implications for recent scholarship in development studies, particularly those that find Kerala to be an exemplar of human development? What may be the shape of contemporary feminist intervention into the knowledge and practice of birth control in Kerala's specific context? The following brief points are attempts to reflect upon each of these questions from within this inquiry.

To begin with, what directions of research does this work point to? First, it is clear that it does not reach into some of the interesting developments of recent decades, such as the gradual spread of the one-child norm, quite visible in contemporary Kerala. Factors that were crucial in the 1970s may have accentuated, transformed, or become effete in the present. Therefore, the issue is not one of merely 'extending' the scope of inquiry in time. Here it may be profitable to caution oneself against the temptation to think in terms of continuity, as if the demographic transition would by itself spiral 'naturally' towards the one-child family. Painstaking analysis that would consider the changes in procreation, sustenance, as well as wide-ranging cultural changes seems quite indispensable here too.

Secondly, though this work does not upturn the belief that popular acceptance of contraception in Kerala was non-coercive, there are indications of forms of indirect pressurizing in the historical sources, which are, however, not pursued at great length. It may be worthwhile to pursue this lead precisely because of the kinds of pressure tactics hinted at seem quite uniquely subtle and capable of escaping scrutiny. For instance, in 1968, K. I. Rajan, a member of the Kerala State Legislative Assembly, asked the health minister whether the government had heard of threats being issued to women workers in plantations that they would be denied work unless they submitted to IUCD insertions (*Proceedings of the Kerala Legislative Assembly* 1969: 618). In 1966, the *Matrubhumi* was reporting complaints from FP workers that those of them who could not mobilize at least five women a day for IUCD insertion were being denied increments (17 October 1966: 4). However, important though this investigation might be, it should by no means be understood that largely underhand tactics garnered the consent for FP here, and that people were soft-bullied into acceptance. Such work may only bring to attention a hitherto less-noticed dimension of the acceptance–generation machinery of the FP establishment, as a necessary qualification of the often over-simplistic adulation for 'voluntary acceptance'.

Related to this is the need for greater attention to the building up of the FP machinery in the state at various levels. From historical sources, it seems quite vital to examine how the hierarchical structure delivering FP services to the people emerged. The tensions within the medical hierarchy were quite visible in the 1960s, for instance in the strikes of FP workers in the lower rungs for better benefits. The first chapter has hinted at how the press also often lamented the inertia of the FP machinery, and showered warm praise on those government functionaries who seemed capable of successfully mobilizing government machinery to the efficient implementation of FP activities. How the building up of the FP machinery was shaped by forms of social control needs to be urgently looked at. For instance, in 1968, the health minister was asked about reports that male acceptors were inconvenienced by the presence of women health personnel during surgeries (*Proceedings of the Kerala State Legislative Assembly* 1969: 618). It would be interesting to follow up this line to explore the ways in which gender relations were shaped and negotiated within the FP establishment. How the machinery was mobilized is thus vitally important in understanding the success of FP in Kerala. A related absence is a full analysis of the changes in the technology of birth control, and the cultural acceptance and 'taming' of technology here (Kaler 2000). The major thrust of this work has been to initiate a broader reflection on social, cultural, and politico–economic processes which came together to produce public consent for FP in Kerala. It is hoped that this will, above all, serve to highlight and justify the need to undertake analysis in all the directions indicated above.

Most important of all, there is an urgent need to combine ethnographic inquiry with historical investigations if we are to capture the specific ways in which particularly situated and endowed social groups and individuals negotiated with, resisted, or subverted the discourse of FP. This may also be necessary to capture regional specificities within Kerala. This work has largely relied upon material focused on southern and central Kerala. Public discourse in Malabar does not seem to have been substantially different. However, as other socio–cultural conditions did differ between Travancore, Cochin, and Malabar, there are likely to be interesting differences in the individual and group negotiations with state-sponsored contraception between these regions.

Secondly, what are the implications of this exploration for the widely-accepted image of Kerala as the near-utopia of human development? This work has concluded that the greater availability and use of contraception in Kerala did not translate into mobility and freedom for women and openness about sexuality. The strong mediating presence of the ideals of individuality rooted in sexual self-disciplining and modern gender, the interests of the patrifocal modern family, and the population-management imperatives of the post-colonial state were pointed out. This would raise the question whether the fairly widespread availability of contraception in Kerala may be interpreted readily to mean that women in Kerala do have the resources for the realization of reproductive rights, and whether the issue is merely one of helping them to convert these resources into capabilities and functionings. It would also ask questions regarding responsibility in making choices: whether the family-oriented reproductive choices that women in Kerala seem to be making can be regarded as 'voluntary'. This work indicates that while resources for family-centred fertility control are widespread in Kerala (the burden of this work has been precisely to trace the historical shaping of the acceptance of these), resources for reproductive health and informed choice without familial pressures simply may not exist. That patriarchal values and socialization processes have equally shaped both the constraints on women's choices—the lack of resources and freedom—and the preferences that underlie their choices is something that this work has sought to focus upon.

It is well known that the Kerala has been ranked first among Indian states in the Human Development Index in 1981, 1991 and 2001 (*National Human Development Report* 2001). The recent Human Development Report on Kerala (HDR) (CDS 2005), clearly admits that notwithstanding the fact that women and men have similar capability sets in many instances, women have been significantly less able to convert their capabilities into useful and desired functionings (CDS 2005: 100–24). The HDR also argues that women's choices are also deeply affected by socio–cultural constraints that direct them to less lucrative, but more 'respectable' kinds of work, and into highly unequal marriages involving dowry payments (CDS 2005: 114–7). Yet there is scarce recognition of the fact that the major burden of fertility reduction lies with the women in Kerala. The strengthening of public services, and measures to combat mental distress, alcoholism, and lifestyle diseases are given priority; reproductive health is completely omitted. Almost mirroring the manner in which popular discourse in Kerala celebrates demographic achievements, but obscures female embodiment and fertility control methods, the HDR elaborates on Kerala's demographic transition and maternal health, but remains silent about gendered patterns of contraceptive use and reproductive health.

While Amartya Sen's 'ethical individualism' in economics has indeed been recognized as being more amenable to concerns regarding gender equality (Robeyns 2001; Agarwal et al. 2006), it also is an open-ended framework quite vulnerable to androcentric interpretations. Indeed, until recently, claims around Kerala's high status in the Human Development Index have implicitly or explicitly relied upon such androcentric versions. These did not exactly ignore the dissimilar conversion rates of women and men with similar capability sets, but scarcely acknowledged that this would seriously qualify Kerala's claim to high levels of human development. Robeyns' point about the conservative application of the capabilities approach rings perfectly true here; here we do have that version which she attributes to 'theorists who are culturally conservative, even if their views on social justice are quite radical' (Robeyns 2001: 16). This is also related to the disciplinary insularity of development-centred disciplines that leads to the survival of naïve ideas within it, which have been clearly discredited elsewhere. For instance, the inability to distinguish between the content and implications of such terms as 'schooling', 'literacy', and 'education' (all three often treated as more or less the same). As Patricia and Roger Jeffrey have pointed out, '... understandings that are commonplace within a critical sociology of education seem not to have impinged on the demographic discussion' (Jeffrey and Jeffrey 1998: 248).

Perhaps the complete silence of issues of gender oppression in reproduction in the HDR relates to a tension within it. There is a certain reluctance to abandon the highly androcentric version of the welfarist human development approach. The significance of gender equality can vary considerably within the welfarist and the neo-liberal versions of the human development approach. The welfarist version would conceive of gender equality in non-instrumental terms, highlighting the expansion of women's life-choices, security, and well-being as empowering and valuable in themselves. The other version, which focuses on the state's role as the provider of human skills to the market, would define gender equality in thoroughly instrumental terms, as a means towards enhancing global competitiveness. In other words, gender equality is found necessary only to exactly that degree to which it enhances the state's global competitiveness. While the recent HDR for Kerala may not be characterized as fully neo-liberal, it does stop short of elaborating a non-androcentric version of the welfarist HD approach. On the one hand, the conclusion of the HDR leans towards viewing gender equality as crucial in tapping 'the energy and talent of young educated women in Kerala, (CDS 2005: 165). On the other hand, its recommendations against dowry, domestic violence, and various public forms of patriarchy (from which women have to be 'protected') stay within the paternalist framework of androcentric welfarism. The neglect of gender oppression in reproduction clearly underlines the latter point. For the expansion of reproductive choices and the struggle against state and patriarchal power upon bodies involve not so much the 'protection' of women, as the widening of their possibilities of resistance and self-strengthening.

Thirdly, what lessons do we learn from the foregoing account for the feminist critique of birth control in Kerala? It may be claimed that this, perhaps, would begin from sustained criticism of the foregrounding of motherly and wifely agency within the discourse of contraception that fixes its meaning as 'family planning'. However, this would also require concerted efforts to create the conditions under which contraception may become a powerful resource to actualize women's bodily autonomy. The preceding chapters have touched upon the shaping of the several constraints that have to be overcome. A good instance would be the techno–scientific language in which sex continues to be discussed here. It was observed in the first chapter that scientific sex education was accepted first in élite intellectual circles, to gradually circulate further in Malayali society, recognized as a superior instrument of regulating sexual desire in individuals. It was also seen that the FPP drew upon this energetically, adopting the scientific–objective language, and setting up non-reciprocal relations between the FP expert and the FP acceptor. The consequences of this hierarchization were also briefly touched upon: in order to speak of sex and sexuality in Malayali society, one has recourse only to either highly alienating and management-oriented scientific language, or that of soft porn, which insists on constructing sex and sexuality in terms of androcentric 'secret pleasures'. Both these languages are equally objectifying, and they perpetuate the sexualization of the female body in their distinct ways. The task ahead, then, is also to create a non-objectifying language in which one may discuss sex and sexuality as everyday matters. Undoubtedly, this is also crucial to disarm the non-reciprocal relations of power that govern sexual practices and contraception. Once stripped of the scientific authority, it becomes much more possible to bring back the focus to user-controlled contraceptive methods, aimed at the reversal of power relations between men and women, and contraceptive provider and user. At the same time, it is important to see that in recent years, a language that links contraception to pleasurable sex and control by the user has been articulated in the promotion of condoms—in the controversial Kamasutra advertisements—which addresses the Indian middle-classes. However, population control, and the language of scientific management that accompanies it, is quite alive and well, now directed all the more forcefully at poor women, 'through methods ranging from (hazardous) injectibles and new anti-pregnancy vaccines, to literacy campaigns. Simple barrier methods will no longer do for them, let alone fertility-awareness based contraceptive practices, which would require the dedicated involvement of the male partner. In sum, the scenario is one in which the 'demand is rather, pleasure for "us" and fertility control for "them".' (John 1998: 387), which must be exposed and challenged.

Another instance would be the constructed harmony between different levels of society implicit in the FP propaganda's projection of birth control as a comprehensive solution to the material and non-material ills of the community, the family, and the individual, mentioned in the third chapter. Such harmony scarcely exists outside such enunciations. Thus what the individual may choose as best for her interests may not necessarily be in harmony with the interests of the collective to which she may belong, or what seems to serve the family's interest best may not seem the best for the larger community of which the family is an intrinsic part. It seems necessary to reverse the strategy of the FP propaganda to ensure that these levels will not be reduced to each other, to the ultimate advantage of one level, that of the nation-state. This will also work as a necessary counter to recent forms of pro-natalism, often directed at women in subtle ways, often from within communities. Indeed, subtler attacks against contraception are currently mounting with or without pro-natalist rhetoric—such as for instance, the conservative sex education programmes circulating in US schools (Rose 2005). In the Malayali context, a climate of intense sexual conservatism prevails, bolstered heavily by conservative neo-religious institutions and ideologies. Concerns are also being expressed about the demographic decline of certain hitherto-prominent communities (for example, Zachariah 2001). The tendency in much popular discourse to implicitly fault the demographic transition as the major cause for much of the social anomie plaguing contemporary Malayali society also needs to be qualified. Such captious criticism only exposes our indolence and unwillingness to search for *collective* solutions to problems such as taking care of a rapidly increasing elderly population, instead of privatized ones, and our failure to shape alternate visions of community, social belonging, and connectedness (Kittay 2006).

An equally important task would be the creation of a politically sensitive, nuanced critique of the patrifocal family in Kerala. While literary fantasies have often depicted situations in which totalitarian regimes deploy advanced eugenics-oriented reproductive technology to weed out the family (like, for instance, in *The Brave New World*), in history, reproductive technologies have been wedded to Western familial values (Posner 2000: 20). As it has been argued in the first and second chapters, contraception in Kerala has been primarily loyal to the aspirations of the nuclear family, and whenever it drew upon the notion of women's control of their bodies, it was in a half-hearted and instrumentalist sense. It can hardly be denied, however, that contraception does hold very real prospects of expanded life-choices for women, which the feminist critique must certainly countenance. Historically, state hostility to contraception was often strongly associated with misogyny and blatant double standards of sexual morality (for instance, in the early twentieth century, Irish Free State, Smith 2004). However, the recent feminist critique of the notion of 'ownership' of one's body that hark to a patriarchal and bourgeois concept of the discrete self that may be subjugated by medical science, population control, or patriarchal kinship systems (Petchesky 1990) must also be seriously taken. Recent work does show that historically, control over embodiment has been granted enormous value in Western culture, and the inability to meet this requirement has been alarmingly disempowering (Twine 2001). The culturalist argument against the Western notion of bodily autonomy, advanced by some feminists (for example, Obermeyer 1994), may not be relevant in the Malayali context, in which Western ideas and practices are hardly 'foreign'. Feminist intervention to reclaim women's bodies should certainly go beyond the task of merely extending developmental idealism, though the tensions between its propositions may well be strategically exploited. Also, a critique of the individualized self needs to be voiced in Malayali society, perhaps more than in any other Indian society (Devika 2002a). Nor is it impossible to link women's struggles for reproductive rights with other struggles—even with those centred around marginal identities (Nelson 2001; Smith 2005).

Importantly, to argue that the critique of reproductive interventions needs to go beyond the liberal notion of autonomy does not necessarily mean that we abandon the area of body politics: one may still problematize the operations of power upon the body without reference to the goal of liberalist bodily autonomy. Nor is it necessary to fall back upon essentialisms, 'discursive' (Fuss 1989) or biological, or be satisfied with theorizing the body as metaphor.[6] Recent feminist reflections indicate that no neat distinction can be drawn between the corporeal and the social, and so what we really have is 'social flesh': the body as a concrete, material space of living which mediates social and cultural relationships (Beasley and Bacchi 2000). This work has foregrounded the extent to which the body is indeed a target of political control and power, constantly subject to public regulation; it has also hinted above that it may also be an area of resistance to such regulation or in other words, a contested area (Harcourt 2004). Feminist geographers have also been increasingly pointing out that the body is a geographical space, which shapes the self rather than a passive container of the self or a blank surface upon which social processes play. The body, they have pointed out, is regarded as a 'private' space which is seen to 'house' sexuality, but which is itself subject to public monitoring (Johnston 1996). Thinking through sexuality, space and social power, it has been pointed out that 'socio–spatial power relations (re)form sexed sites and, in turn, the (re)constitution of places sexes bodies' (Browne 2004: 335). Acknowledging that body-space does shape us in crucial ways means that the struggles over the body need to be necessarily more than simply over the ownership of sexuality. The question, then, is how we may challenge the fixing of the body into specific places, and not merely about whether the 'owner' of the body wishes it or not.

Later eco–feminist positions have been sceptical of both the liberal call to transcend the 'limitations' of the body, and the earlier eco-feminist identification of women's bodies with nature and their idealization of mothering (Roach 1991). They have also pointed out that a distinction should be drawn between '... reclaiming one's sense of embodiment from others (for example, contraception and abortion) and adopting an actual, highly disciplined and mastering approach to one's embodiment' (Twine 2001: 34). It seems important for the feminist reclaiming of contraception to take on board Richard Twine's observation that 'the human body is inherently fragile or vulnerable ... Moreover, we should take into account the agency of our embodiment. For instance, human bodies may produce side-effects to animal-tested medicines, invasive cosmetic surgeries and other ill-thought out technologies that forget this fragility' (Twine 2001: 51). Taking this seriously will mean that we remain wary of individual choices that violate the 'agency of embodiment'. For instance, when women who are desperately poor, abused, remain unhealthy due to the lack of real choices—

who have no other means of improving the unfavourable life conditions within which they find themselves trapped—opt for sterilization as a way of improving the conditions of their lives, this cannot be glibly read off as a sign of 'conscious choice' or 'independent agency'.[7]

The importance of effective birth control in the history of the expansion of women's rights is unmistakable: we have many accounts that describe the struggles of the early feminists for birth control around the world in the twentieth century (for instance, Fraser 1999). The question, however, is not whether we accept or reject reproductive technologies as such, but rather how we can remain alert to the specific operations of power in local contexts.[8] Thus, even as we struggle for self-determination against more immediate sources of oppression that seeks to appropriate women's reproductive capacities in ways that harm women, it is important that we stay alert to equally pervasive and insidious forms of power that may, however, appear more distant—such as the global and national imperatives of population control—which operate precisely through the discourse of 'women's autonomy', or, to disguised forms of eugenics that caters to 'consumers' choices' (Daniels and Golden 2004). It seems, on one hand, important to constantly question the narratives that shape our notions of self-sufficiency, autonomy, and the like, which circulate ubiquitously in and through popular media while on the other hand, efforts at expanding the range of choices also appear vital. Motherhood, for instance, is hardly an 'option' in Malayali society, in the sense that it is tied to the social pressure to marry, set up a home, and maintain it. It may be possible to think about ways of turning motherhood into an actually pleasurable option for women, by radically redefining it, cutting it loose from its present moorings in the notion of the individualized, disciplined, and productive self, and in the privatized, insular space of the modern family.

Notes

1 Personal conversation with Dr Uma Mohandas, Kollam.

2 This thesis has been advanced in Alaka M. Basu, 'Birth Control by Assetless Workers in Kerala: The Possibility of a Poverty Induced Fertility Transition',

Development and Change, 17, 2, 1986, 265–82. A study conducted by the Demographic Research Centre of the University of Kerala revealed that 43.33 per cent of the sterilized persons in 1971–2 were unskilled workers; another study of the FP acceptors of the mass sterilization camp at Thiruvananthapuram (of June 1972) observed that overwhelming significance was being given to remuneration in cash by the acceptors (G.S. Nair and P.G. Nair, *Selected Studies on Population and Family Welfare Programme,* vol. ii, Demographic Research Centre, Thiruvananthapuram, University of Kerala, 1978, 31; 154).

[3] It will certainly be pointed out here that a range of written sources, especially biographies and autobiographies from mid-twentieth century Kerala, contain accounts of young sons and husbands setting aside their domestic responsibilities and plunging into nationalist or communist politics. I would however like to point out that such politics often appealed precisely to the sanctity of home life and domestic obligations for self-justification. These figures, then, are represented as selfless heroes who sacrifice their (domestic) interests and loves for the well-being of other people/other families. Several such instances may be culled from leftist popular theatre of the twentieth century. In P.J. Antony's hugely popular play *Inquilabinte Makkal* (The children of revolution), Francis, the pro-Communist character, raises this point to convince his frustrated unemployed friend of the need for socialism: ' Parents raise and educate their children in the hope that they will protect the parents in their old age... So when the expectations of parents regarding their children are shattered, the very desires of their life are shattered ... it is this system that must be opposed. Family relations are being shattered. That even our dearest ties have to be dependent on money! What a pitiable situation! ... Only if Man is economically free will love exist in its truest form.' *Inquilabinte Makkal* [1954], Kottayam, SPSS, 1980, 26.

[4] While much more research is certainly necessary to answer the question why we find a sharp fall in the male sterilization rate after 1976–7, the state's use of sterilization during the Emergency may have indeed revealed how sterilization, hitherto projected as ensuing from the benevolence of the state, could be well part of its coercive machinery. However, looking at the figures for the 1970s, we find that vasectomies exceeded the figure for 1971–2 (the year of the mass sterilization camps) only once, in 1976, while tubectomies register a more or less steady rise through the 1970s. In 1973–4 and 1975–6, the number of vasectomies fell to 14,751 and 18,466, respectively, to rise again in the following two years, and then to decrease steadily thereafter (N.M. Beevi, 'An Evaluation of Family Welfare Programme in Kerala, India, 1992', *in* G.N. Rao (ed.) *Family Planning: The Afro-Asian Scenarios*, Centre for Development Studies, Thiruvananthapuram, 1999, 241). This indicates that even the Emergency excesses may have left domestic ideologies quite unshaken in Kerala; the fall in 1973 and 1974 could have been partly a reaction to frequent failure of vasectomy, much reported and lampooned in the press, following which FP propaganda was doubled. The impact of the shift in the national programme towards women

post-Emergency and the coming of new surgical techniques may have aided the subsequent turn towards tubectomies.

[5] I am grateful to P.K. Michael Tharakan for pointing out to me that the 'mass' programmes initiated by the left, and taken forward by successive governments since the early 1970s, were saturated with the ideology of modern domesticity and served to bolster rather than question the overwhelming importance granted to familial existence in modern Malayali society, and that there was little in these that would prompt citizens to demand a rejuvenated sense of the public.

[6] It has been pointed out that radical constructivist positions that problematize notions of 'nature' and 'body' as discursive constructions are sensitive to history and cultural difference, but often function as 'discursive essentialisms' that 'merely reproduces the modernist *and* anthropocentric framework of the culture/nature dualism, granting more value and explanatory power to culture ... A position of radical social constructionism in relation to nature and bodies defiantly shifts notions of essence firmly into the realm of 'culture' and 'mind'. Thus, with not a scent of irony, such postmodernist conceptualization actually completes the modernist project of mastery.' R.T. Twine, 'Ma(r)king Essence: Ecofeminism and Embodiment', *Ethics and Environment,* 6, 2, 2001, 35.

[7] Johanna Schoen, in her study of the state's denial of elective sterilization services to poor or ill women in North Carolina, argues that 'Some poor women and women of color actively sought sterilization. Rather than being the victims of coercive eugenic policies, they used those policies and programs for their own ends' (J. Schoen, 'Between Choice and Coercion: Women and the Politics of Sterilization in North Carolina 1929–1975, *Journal of Women's History,* 13, 1, 2001, 133). However, this is to play down the fact that this was also the only way open to those women, that offered any hope of changing their lives. Women's 'agency', in this case, rests clearly upon the violation of the agency of their embodiment.

[8] Anthony Giddens's claim about the effects of the separation of sexuality and reproduction through contraception, that it leads to 'plastic sexuality' and 'confluent love' that opens new, positive possibilities in male-female relationships comes to mind here (Anthony Giddens, *The Transformation of Intimacy*, Cambridge, Polity Press, 1992). However, Hera Cook's criticism of Giddens is vitally important: she points out the contraception by itself cannot bring about these possibilities, and 'Giddens's "pure" relationships are not because only the exceptional woman earns enough to perform as a self-reflective, financially self-sufficient worker and responsible risk-taker.' Hera Cook, 'The English Sexual Revolution: Technology and Social Change', *History Workshop Journal,* 59, 2005, 124.

Bibliography

Legislative Assembly Proceedings

Cochin Legislative Council Proceedings vol. vi, 1–15, 1934.

Proceedings of the Travancore Sree Mulam Assembly vol. xii–ii, 1939, vol. xx, 1945, vol. xxv, 1946, vol. xxvi, 1946a.

Proceedings of the Travancore–Cochin Legislative Assembly, vol. i, 16–33, 1951, vol. iii, 1–2, 1952.

Proceedings of the Kerala State Legislative Assembly vol. I, 1958, vol. vii, 1960, vol. ix, 1961, vol. xxi, 1968, vol. xxii, 1969, Vol. xxii, 1969.

Government Reports

Travancore Administration Report, 1865–66.

Report of the Malabar Marriage Commission [1891], Lawrence Asylum Press, Madras.

Report of the Ezhava Law Committee, Government of Travancore, Thiruvananthapuram, 1919.

Report of the Travancore Unemployment Enquiry Committee, Government of Travancore, Thiruvananthapuram, 1928.

Report of the Travancore Educational Reforms Committee, Government of Travancore, Thiruvananthapuram, 1933.

Report of the Beggar Relief Committee, Government of Cochin, Cochin, 1944.

Report of the Committee for Evaluation of Family Welfare Programme (Kerala), Government of Kerala, Thiruvananthapuram, 1978.

National Human Development Report 2001, Planning Commission, Government of India, New Delhi, 2002.

Newspapers and Periodicals

Selected volumes/issues of

Aryakeralam, 1935.

Arogyam, 1932–6.
Deepam, 1933.
Deshabhimani, 1952–70.
Janayugam Weekly, 1958, 74; 1956–71 (Annual Numbers).
Jayakeralam, 1958.
Kaumudi Weekly, 1951–8.
Kerala Kaumudi, 1960–72.
Kutumbapatrika, 1934–5.
Lakshmibhayi, 1913.
Mahila, 1930–6.
Matrubhumi, 1950–72; 1930–6.
Malayala Manorama, 1958–72; 1906; 1910.
Matrubhumi Weekly, 1960–5.
Malayala Manorama Weekly, 1948–48.
Malayalarajyam, 1952–69.
Mangalodayam, 1930.
M.N. Nair Masika, 1936–8.
Navasarasan, 1935.
Nazrani Deepika, 1929–60.
Nazrani Deepika Weekly, 1951–2.
Rasikan, 1934.
Service, 1926.
Stree, 1933.
Swadeshabhimani, 1924–5.
Swajanaranjini, 1934.
Unny Nambutiri, 1925.
Vanitaratnam, 1928–35.
Vivekodayam, 1930–1.
Yuvachaitanyam, 1933.
Yuvakeralam, 1939.

Select Editorials

Nazrani Deepika, 'Tiruvitamkoorile Nelkrishi' (Rice farming in Travancore), 14 Feb. 1936, 2.

——, 'Sadhukkalkku Potuve Colony Erppeduttanam' (The poor must be rehabilitated in colonies), 28 June 1939, 2.

——, 'Yachakparasnam' (The beggar problem), 18 Feb. 1941, 2.

——, 'Bhakshanavishayattil Svayamparyaptata' (Self-reliance in food-matters), 22 Feb. 1941, 4.

——, 'Onakkalam' (The Onam season), 2 Sept. 1941, 2.

——, 'Samudayasanghatanakal' (Community movements), 14 Sept. 1949, 2.

——, 'Pratividhi Entu?' (What is the solution?), 24 June 1952, 2.

——, 'Janaperuppam' (Population boom), 11 April 1953, 2.

Desabhimani, 'Janapperuppathinte Karyam' (The matter of population boom), 18 June 1953, 2.

Nazrani Deepika, 'Nammude State Budget' (Our State budget) 19 July 1954, 2.

——, 'Kutumbasamvidhanam' (Family Planning), 15 April 1958, 2.

Malayala Manorama, 'Keralattinte Vyavasayavalkkaranam' (Industrialization of Kerala), 20 Nov. 1958, 2.

Malayalarajyam, 'Kutumbasamvidhanam' (Family Planning), 13 Dec. 1958, 2.

Malayala Manorama, 'Keralavum Ghanavyavasayangalum' (Kerala and heavy industries), 15 Jan. 1959, 2.

——, 'Keralattile Bhakshyolppadanavikasanam' (Development of food production in Kerala), 19 March 1960, 2.

Nazrani Deepika, 'Dakshina Kanara Malayalikal' (Malayalis in South Kanara), 8 Oct. 1960, 2.

——, 'Mysore Governmentum Malayali Karshakarum' (The Mysore government and Malayali farmers), 11 Oct. 1960, 2.

Malayala Manorama, 'Kendravum Keralavum', 14 Sept. 1960, 2.

——, 'Keralam Anukarikkenda Vyavasayavalkkarana Matruka' (Models of industrialization Kerala ought to emulate), 14 Oct. 1960, 4.

Kerala Kaumudi, 'Vargeeyatayum Mukhyamantrimarute Sammelanavum' (Communal politics and the chief ministers' conference), *Kerala Kaumudi,* 15 Aug. 1961, 2.

Matrubhumi, 'Keralattinte Vikasanam' (Kerala's development), 27 April 1962, 2.

Malayala Manorama, 'Dr. Lokanathante Report, 1 May 1962, 2.

——, 'Sarkar Vanangalile Kutiyettakkar' (Migrants in government forests), 15 Jan. 1963, 2.

——, 'Kutiyetta Paddhati' (Plan for migration), 30 Jan. 1963, 2.

Malayalarajyam, 'Lokarogyavum Janasankhyaprasnavum' (People's health and the population problem), 9 April 1963, 2.
Malayala Manorama, 'High Rangeile Kutiyozhippikkal' (Eviction in the high ranges), 27 April 1963, 2.
Malayalarajyam, 'Keralattile Kudumbasootranam' (Family Planning in Kerala), 21 Dec. 1963, 2.
——, 'Janapperuppam' (Population boom), 26 Aug. 1964, 1.
Matrubhumi, 'Kutumbasootranam' (Family Planning), 19 Dec. 1965, 4.
——, 'Aaru Pizhachu?' (Who is at fault?'), 30 Dec. 1965, 4.
——, 'Nalaunso?' (Four ounces?!), 7 Jan. 1966, 4.
Malayala Manorama, 'Tainan-3 Krishi' (Cultivation of Tainan-3), 6 May 1966, 2.
——, 'Vivekashoonyamaya Prakshobhanam' (Imprudent protest), 2 Nov. 1966, 2.
Matrubhumi, 'Nammude Gati' (Our fate), 31 July 1966, 4.
——, 'Keralttinte Nalampaddhati' (The Fourth Plan in Kerala), 7 Sept. 1966, 6.
——, 'Keralattinte Sampattu' (The wealth of Kerala), 13 Nov. 1966, 4.
——, 'Oru Kroora Vinodam' (A cruel joke), 17 Nov. 1966, 6.
Kerala Kaumudi, 'Vivahaprayam' (Age of marriage), 7 Jan. 1967, 2.
Matrubhumi, 'Arkku Vottu Cheyyanam?' (Whom to vote for?), 14 Feb. 1967, 3.
——, 'Videshanaanayam Kondu Kasarth' (Bravado over foreign exchange), 9 June 1967, 4.
Malayala Manorama 'Vazhipizhaccha Bhakshyanayam' (Mistaken food policy), 19 June 1967, 2.
Kerala Kaumudi, 'Kutumbasootranam' (Family Planning) 21 June 1967, 2.
——, 'Kerala Governmentum Kutumbasootranavum' (The Kerala government and FP), 30 June 1967, 2.
——, 'Janasankhyaaniyantranam' (Population control), 5 Aug. 1967, 2.
Matrubhumi, 'Keralattinte Durgati' (Kerala's ill-Fate), 8 Aug. 1967, 4.

Kerala Kaumudi, 'Vyavasayavalkkaranam' (Industrialization), 28 Dec. 1967, 2.

——, 'Uttarendyaile Malayalikal' (Malayalis in North India), 25 May 1968, 2.

——, 'Verittunilkkal' (Separatism), 21 May 1968, 2.

Malayalarajyam, 'Kutumbasootranam' (Family Planning), 29 Nov. 1968, 2.

Kerala Kaumudi, 'Kendra Government Pratikkootil' (Central government in the dock), 20 Feb. 1969, 2.

Malayala Manorama, 'Keralam Madrasine Kandu Paddhikkumo?' (Will Kerala learn from Madras?), 2 July 1969, 4.

Kerala Kaumudi, 'Tozhilillaima' (Unemployment), 20 July 1969, 2.

Matrubhumi, 'Gudalloorile Kutiyirakku' (Evictions in Gudalloor), 19 Sept. 1969, 4.

——, 'Pottitterikkunna Janasankhyaprasnam' (The problem of exploding population), 7 Dec. 1969, 4.

——, 'Samtriptakutumbam' (Contented family), 7 Jan. 1970, 2.

——, 'Tozhilillaatta Engineermar' (Unemployed engineers), 5 March 1970, 4.

——, 'Enthinu Karayunnu?' (Why Cry?), 7 May 1970, 3.

——, 'Parihasikkarutu, Apamanikkarutu' (Do not mock, do not insult), 5 June 1970, 4.

Kerala Kaumudi, 'Kutumbasootranam' (Family Planning), 12 July 1970, 2.

Matrubhumi, 'Janaperuppa Pratirodha Yajnam' (*Yajna* against population boom), 22 Dec. 1970, 4.

Kerala Kaumudi 'SNDP Yogam', 16 Dec. 1970, 2.

Matrubhumi 'Garbhacchidram' (Abortion), 2 June 1971, 2.

Kerala Kaumudi, 'Gudalloorile Kutiyirakku' (Eviction in Gudalloor), 10 Sept. 1971, 2.

Books and Theses

Abdulkhadar, Vakkom M. (1947): *Vicharavedi* [Collection of essays], Udaya Publishing, Punalur.

Agarwal, Bina, Jane Humphries, Ingrid Robeyns (eds.) (2006): *Capabilities, Freedom, and Equality: Amartya Sen's Work from a*

Gender Perspective, Oxford University Press, New Delhi.

Aiyar, C.P. Ramaswamy, (1945): *Selections from the Writings and Speeches of Sachivottama Sir. C.P. Ramaswamy Aiyar*, Government Press, Thiruvananthapuram.

Amma, B. Kalyani. (1968): *Ormayil Ninnu* [memoirs], K. Gomati Amma (ed.), Sahitya Pravartaka Sahakarana Sangham, Kottayam.

Amma, Kochattil Kalyanikutty, (1991): *Pathikayum Vazhiyoratte Manideepangalum* (The Traveller and the Wayside Lamps (autobiography)), Thrissur.

Amma, Saraswati, K. (1955): *Premabhajanam* (The Beloved [novel]), Sahitya Pravartaka Sahakarana Sangham, Kottayam.

Antony, P.J. [1954] (1980) *Inquilabinte Makkal* (The Children of the Revolution) Sahitya Pravartaka Sahakarana Sangham, Kottayam.

Arunima, G. (2003): *There Comes Papa: Colonialism and the Transformation of Matriliny in Kerala, Malabar c.1850–1940*, Orient Longman, Hyderabad.

Babu, I.V. (2001): *Keraleeyanavoddhanavum Nambutirimarum* (Kerala's Renaissance and the Nambutiris), Sahitya Pravartaka Sahakarana Sangham, Kottayam.

Balakrishnan, Venganoor. (2000): *Balaramapuram G. Raman Pillai* [biography], Navasakti Books, Thiruvananthapuram.

Banerjee. D. (1971): *Family Planning in India: A Critique and a Perspective*, People's Publishing House, New Delhi.

——, (1985): *Health and Family Planning Services in India*, Lok Paksh, New Delhi.

Basu, Alaka M., Peter Aaby (eds.) (1988): *The Methods and Uses of Anthropological Demography*, Clarendon Press, Oxford.

Bhaskaran, T. (Comp). (2000): *Sree Narayanaguru Vaighari*, Kunnattunad SNDP Union, Perumbavoor.

Bhattatiripad, V.T. (1988): *Karmavipakam* [Autobiography], Best Books, Changanashery.

Blandford, Augusta (1904): *The Land of the Conch Shell*, Church of England Zenana Missionary Society, London.

Corea, Genea. (1985): *The Mother Machine: Reproductive Technologies from Artificial Insemination to Artificial Wombs*, Harper and Row, New York.

Cowen, M.P, and R.W. Shenton. (1996): *Doctrines of Development*, Routledge, London.

Chandrasekharan, M.R. (1999): *Keralattile Purogamanasahityaprasthanatinte Charitram* (The History of the Progressive Writers' Movement in Kerala), Olive Books, Kozhikode.

Centre for Development Studies (2005): *Human Development Report 2005: Kerala*, Government of Kerala, Thiruvananthapuram.

Coale, A.J. and E.M. Hoover (1958): *Population Growth and Economic Development in Low Income Countries*, Princeton University Press, Princeton, New Jersey.

Correa, S, and R. Reichman (1994): *Population and Reproductive Rights: Feminist Perspectives From the South*, Kali for Women, New Delhi.

Damodaran, K. (1952): *Marxisavum Kutumbajeevitavum* (Marxism and Family Life), Thiruvananthapuram.

Damodaran, K. (1947): *Omana* (novel), Indira Publications, Thiruvananthapuram.

Daniels, C. (1993): *At Women's Expense*, Harvard University Press, Cambridge, Massachusetts.

Davis, Kingsley (1951): *The Population of India and Pakistan*, Russell and Russell, New York.

den Uyl, Marion, (1995): *Invisible Barriers: Gender, Caste and Kinship in a Southern Indian Village*, International Books, Utrecht.

Devika, J. (ed. and trans.) (2005): *Her-Self: Early Writings on Gender by Malayali Women*, Stree, Kolkata.

——, (2007): *En-Gendering Individuals: The Language of Re-forming in Early Twentieth Century Keralam,* Orient Longman, Hyderabad.

Donaldson, P.J. (1990): *Nature Against Us: The United States and the World Population Crisis 1965–1980*, University of North Carolina Press, Chapel Hill.

Erwer, Monica (2003): *Challenging the Gender Paradox: Women's Collective Agency in the Transformation of Kerala Politics*, Department of Peace and Development Studies, Goteborg University, Goteborg.

Escobar, Arturo (1995): *Encountering Development: The Making and Unmaking of the Third World,* Princeton University Press, Princeton, New Jersey.

Eysteinsson, Astradur (1990): *The Concept of Modernism*, Cornell University Press, Cornell.

Feldman-Savelsberg, Pamela (1999): *Plundered Kitchens, Empty Wombs: Threatened Reproduction and Identity in the Cameroon Grassfields*, University of Michigan Press, Ann Arbor.

Ferguson, James (1990): *The Anti-politics Machine: Development, Depoliticization and Bureaucratic Power in Lesotho*, University of Minnesota Press, Minneapolis.

Foucault, Michel. (1978): *The History of Sexuality, Vol. I: An Introduction*, Penguin, Harmondsworth.

Furedi, Frank (1997): *Population and Development: A Critical Introduction*, Polity Press, Oxford.

Fuss, Diana (1989): *Essentially Speaking: Feminism, Nature and Difference*, Routledge, London.

Frankel, Francine R. (1971): *India's Green Revolution: Economic Gains and Political Costs*, Princeton University Press, Princeton.

Gandhi Grandhalayalam (1955): *Lingavijnanam: Balabodhini* (Sex Education for Boys), Thrissur.

——, (1955): *Lingavijnanam: Balikabodhini* (Sex Education for Girls), Thrissur.

——, (1955) *Purushanmarude Laingikaroganagal* (Sexual Diseases of Men), Thrissur.

George, K.C. (1985) *Ente Jeevitayatra* (The Journey of My Life (autobiography)), Mavelikkara, Kerala.

Giddens, Anthony (1992): *The Transformation of Intimacy: Sexuality, Love and Eroticism in Modern Societies*, Polity Press, Cambridge.

Gopalan, A.K. (1980): *Ente Jeevita Katha* (The Story of My Life (autobiography)), Deshabhimani, Thiruvananthapuram.

Gopalan, Ettumanoor (1993): *Dewer Enna Karmadheeran* (biography), Dewer Smaraka Samiti, Kochi.

Gordon, Linda (1976): *Woman's Body, Woman's Right: A Social History of Birth Control in America*, Grossman, New York.

Government of India (2003): *Family Welfare Yearbook, 2001*,

Ministry of Health and Family Welfare, New Delhi.

Greenhalgh, Susan (ed.) (1995) *Situating Fertility: Anthropology and Demographic Inquiry*, Cambridge University Press, Cambridge.

Gulati, L. (1981): *Profiles in Female Poverty: A Study of Five Poor Working Women in Kerala*, Hindustan Publishing Corporation, New Delhi.

Gupta. A. (1999): *Post-colonial Developments: Agriculture in the Making of Modern India*, Oxford University Press, New Delhi.

Hatch, D. Spencer (1932): *Up from Poverty in Rural Travancore*, Oxford University Press, Bombay.

Heller, Patrick (1999): *The Labor of Development: Workers and the Transformation of Capitalism in Kerala, India*, Cornell University Press, New York.

Jamal (1975): *Kunhusahib* (biography of P.K. Kunhu), Kochi.

Jeffrey, Robin (2003): *Politics, Women and Well-being: How Kerala became a 'Model'*, Oxford University Press, New Delhi.

——, (1976): *The Decline of Nayar Dominance*, Sussex University Press, London.

Jose, C.H. (1975): *Dambatyajeevitattiloode* (Through Marital Life), Janata Publications, Tevara.

——, (1970): *Achchanum Ammayum Akumbol* (Becoming Father and Mother), Janata Publications, Tevara.

——, (1971): *Premavum Samarppanavum* (Love and Dedication), Janata Publications, Tevara.

Joseph, Annie, (1954): *Ee Kattukal Ninakkullatanu* (These Letters are for You (articles)), Kottayam.

Joseph, C.H. (1972): *Matrutvavum Manasakhsiyum* (Motherhood and Conscience), Brothers Book Centre, Thrissur.

——, (1969): *Valarchayude Prasnangal* (The Problems of Growing), Janata, Kochi.

Kalappura, Chackochan, (1972): *Valarchayum Manasatravum* (Growth and Psychology), Janata Publications, Tevara.

Kannan, K.P. (1988): *Of Rural Proletarian Struggles: Mobilisation and Organisation of Rural Workers in South-West India*, Oxford University Press, New Delhi.

Kertzer, David I. (1993): *Sacrificed for Honor: Italian Infant*

Abandonment and the Politics of Reproductive Control, Beacon Press, Boston.

Kesavan, C. (1953) *Jeevitasamaram,*Vol I (autobiography), Sahitya Pravartaka Sahakarana Sangham, Kottayam.

Kooiman, Dick. (1995) *Communities and Electorates: A Comparative Discussion of Communalism in Colonial India*, Comparative Asian Studies 16, VU University Press, Amsterdam.

Krishnankutty, M. (1961): *Chati, Vanchana, Kritrimam* (collection of humorous essays), Kottayam.

Kumar, S. Krishna. (1971): *The Story of the Ernakulam Experiment in Family Planning*, Government of Kerala, Thiruvananthapuram.

Kunhappa, Ch. (1981) *Smaranakal Matram* (autobiography), Kozhikode.

Kunhikrishnan, V.V. (1996): *Keraleeyanum Karshaka Prasthanavum* (Keraleeyan and the Peasants' Movement in Kerala), Deshabhimani Publications, Thiruvananthapuram.

Kurien, M. (1958): *Aanum Pennumayi Avare Srishticchu* (They Were Created Male and Female), Kerala Student Christian Movement, Kottayam.

Kurup, Parameshwara, Koyippalli. (1928): *Vivaharangam* (The Arena of Marriage), Kozhikode.

Lindberg, Anna, (2001): *Experience and Identity: A Historical Account of Class, Caste and Gender among the Cashew Workers of Kerala, 1930–2000*, Lund, Department of History, University of Lund, Lund.

Lewis, Jane (1980): *The Politics of Motherhood: Child and Maternal Welfare in England, 1900–1939*, London, Croon Helm.

Mahadevan, K, and M. Sumangala (1987): *Social Development, Cultural Change and Fertility Decline: A Study of Fertility Change in Kerala*, Sage Publications, New Delhi.

Mammen, P. M. (1981): *Communalism vs. Communism: A Study of the Socio-Religious Communities* and *Political Parties in Kerala, 1892–1970*, Minerva, Calcutta.

Manikkathan, D. (1972): *Kutumbaramam* (The Garden of the Family), Janata Publications, Tevara.

——, (1973): *Dambatyaprasnangal* (Problems of Married Life), Janata Publications, Tevara.

Mannadiyar, V.I. (1949) [1924]: *Kamalam* (novel), P.K. Brothers, Kozhikode.

Marchand, Roland. (1985): *Advertising and the American Dream: Making Way for Modernity, 1920–1940*, University of California Press, Berkeley.

Mathew, P.M. (1968): *Ningalude Jeevita Prasnangal* (Problems of Your Life) [psychological essays], Kottayam.

Mayer, A.C. (1952): *Land and Society in Malabar*, Oxford University Press, London.

McLaren, Angus (1990): *A History of Contraception: From Antiquity to the Present Day*, Blackwell, Oxford.

Menon, O. Chandu (1991) [1889]: *Indulekha* (novel), D.C Books, Kottayam.

Menon, Dilip, M. (1994): *Caste, Nationalism and Communism in South India: Malabar, 1900–1948*, Cambridge University Press, Cambridge.

Menon, A. Gopala (1924): *Samudayollkkarsham* (The Progress of Society), S.R. Book Depot, Thiruvananthapuram.

Menon, P.K.K. (1972): *The History of the Freedom Movement in Kerala* vol. ii. Government of Kerala, Thiruvananthapuram.

Menon, T.K. Krishna, (1948): *Lekhanamala*, Sri Rama Vilasom Press, Kollam.

Menon, K. Narayana, (1929): *Samyogachintaratnam,* Mangalodayam, Thrissur.

——, (1930): *Dambatyarahasyam* (The Secrets of Marriage), Jnanasagaram, Thrissur.

Menon, Nalappattu Narayana (1938): *Ratisamrajyam,* Matrubhumi Publications, Kozhikode.

Menon, Padoo, Komattil [1892] (1985): *Lakshmikesavam, in* P.V. George Irumbayam (ed.), *Nalu Novelukal,* Kerala Sahitya Akademi, Thrissur, 125–218.

Menon, K.P.S. (1971): *Atmakatha* (autobiography), Sahitya Pravartaka Sahakarana Sangham, Kottayam.

Menon, Ramankutty, Kizhakkepattu. [1892] (1985): *Parangodiparinayam* (novel), *in* P.V. George Irumbayam (ed.), *Nalu Novelukal,* Kerala Sahitya Akademi, Thrissur, 219–70.

Menon, Puthezhattu Raman, (1959): *Kazhchappadukal,* vol.i (autobiography), Thrissur.

Menon, V.R. (1973): *Matrubhumiyute Charitram* (The History of *Matrubhumi*), Matrubhumi Publications, Kozhikode.

Menon, V.R. Dr (1970): *Ina Cherumbol* (While Mating), Mangalodayam, Thrissur.

Menon, V.T. Sankunni, and Vidwan V.M. Govinda Menon (1933): *Paurusha Prabhavam*, Norman Printing Bureau, Calicut.

Myrdal, G.K. (1968): *Asian Drama: An Inquiry into the Poverty of Nations,* vols. ii and iii, Penguin, Harmondsworth.

Nair, K. Bhaskaran, (1951): *Dhanyavaadam* [collection of essays], Matrubhumi, Kozhikode.

Nair, Bhaskaran, Tottappalli, (1947): *Bharati Athava Parajayangal* (novel), Vidyarambham Press, Alleppey.

Nair, Cheruvalathu Chathu (1988) [1890]: *Meenakshi* (novel), Kerala Sahitya Akademi, Thrissur.

Nair, G.S, and P.G. Nair (1978): *Selected Studies on Population and Family Welfare Programme,* vol. ii, Demographic Research Centre, Bureau of Economics and Statistics, Thiruvananthapuram.

Nair, N.J. (1940): *A Plea for a New Outlook in Travancore*, Kerala Bandhu Press, Singapore.

Nair, K. Kannan. (1989): *Atmakatha* (autobiography), Matrubhumi, Kozhikode.

Nair, Karunakaran E.A. (1968): *Njan Engane Undayi?* (How was I Born?), Sahitya Pravartaka Sahakarana Sangham, Kottayam.

Nair, Punalur Sudarshanan, (1970) *Premavum Dambatyavum* (Love and Marriage), Kottayam.

Nair, M. Shreekantan (1947): *Aikyakeralam* (United Kerala), Keralabhoomi Books, Thrissur.

Nambutiri Family Regulation Committee Report (1925): Yogakshemam, Thrissur.

Nambutiri, Neelakantan (1929): *Putrolpadanavidhi*, Mangalodayam Press, Thrissur.

Nambutiripad, Kanippayur Sankaran. (1963): *Ente Smaranakal,* vol. i (Memoirs), Panchangom Press, Thrissur.

Nanu, Omalloor, K.V. (1960): *Gramasaubhagyam* (Prosperity of the Village), Kottayam.

Narayanan, C.R. (1960) [1952]: *Janananiyantranam* (Birth Control), Sahitya Pravartaka Sahakarana Sangham, Kottayam.

Narikkuzhi, (1954): *Kutumbathinu Nere* (Against the Family)[1952] S.H. League, Aluva.

Nossiter, T. (1982): *Communism in Kerala: A Study in Political Adaptation*, University of California, Berkeley.

Osella, Caroline, and Filippo Osella (2000): *Social Mobility in Kerala: Modernity in Conflict*, Pluto Press, London.

Ouwerkerk, Louise, (1994): *No Elephants for the Maharajah: Social and Political Change in the Princely State of Travancore (1921–1947)*, Manohar Publications, New Delhi.

Padmadas, S.S.P. (2000): *Intergenerational Transmission of Health: Reproductive Health of Mother and Child Survival In Kerala, India*, thesis, Amsterdam, Thela.

Panikar, P.G. K, T.N. Krishnan N. Krishnaji. (1978): *Population Growth and Agricultural Development: A Case Study of Kerala*, UNFPA, FAO, Rome.

Panikker, M. K. (1954) *Malloor: Oru Matruka Jeevitam* (biography), Thiruvananthapuram.

Parayil, Govindan (ed.) (2000), *Kerala: The Development Experience*, Zed Books, London and New York.

Pateman, Carole (1989) *The Disorder of Women*, Polity Press, Cambridge.

Pavanan (pseudonym), (1967): *Keralam Engane Jeevikkunnu*? (How does Kerala Live), Sahitya Pravartaka Sahakarana Sangham, Kottayam.

Petchesky, R. (1990): *Abortion and Women's Choice: The State, Sexuality and Reproductive Freedom*, North Eastern University Press, Boston.

Peetambaran, K. (1969): *Kutumbasootranam* (Family Planning), Sahitya Pravartaka Sahakarana Sangham, Kottayam.

Pillai, Balakrishna A. (1989): *Kesariyude Mukhaprasangangal* (editorials), D.C Books, Kottayam.

Pillai, Gopala K. (1954): *Pulakolgaman Athava Iruttum Velichavum* (novel), Kollam, Sreeramavilasam Press.

Pillai, Gopalakrishna, Kidangoor A. (Comp.) (1977): *Mannattinte Sampoorna Kritikal* (The Complete Works of Mannath

Padmanabhan), Vidyarthimitram Press, Kottayam, 1977.

Pillai, G.R. (1936): *Grammenapunarudharanam* (Village Reconstruction), Thiruvananthapuram.

Pillai, Narayana, Amshi. (1931–2): *Mahatma Gandhiyude Atmasamyamanam* (Self-Control as Practiced by Mahatma Gandhi), Thiruvananthapuram.

Pillai, V.R. Parameshwaran (1974) *Aa Ezhupatu Varshangal* (autobiography), Thiruvananthapuram.

Pillai, T.K. Velu [1940] (1996): *Travancore Manual,* vol. iii, Kerala State Gazetteers Department, Thiruvananthapuram.

Pisharady, Govinda, Cherukad. (1971): *Devalokam* (novel), Deshabhimani Publications, Thiruvananthapuram.

——, (1984) *Jeevitapata,* (The Path of Life) (autobiography) Deshabhimani, Thiruvanantapuram.

Ponnookkara, Louis (1979): *Avan Valarunnu* (He is Growing), Janata Publications, Tevara.

——, (1979a): *Aval Valarunnu* (She is Growing), Janata Publications, Tevara.

Puthenkalam, J. (1977): 'Marriage and Family in Kerala with Special References to the Matrilineal Castes', George Kurien (ed.), *Journal of Comparative Family Studies Monograph Series,* University of Calgary, Alberta.

Ramanathaiyer, Sundar, and Stewart Macpherson, (2000): *Social Development in Kerala: Illusion or Reality?*, SOAS Studies on Development Geography, Aldershot, Ashgate, Singapore.

Rammohan, K.T. (1996): 'Material Processes and Developmentalism: Interpreting Economic Change in Colonial Tiruvitamkoor 1800–1945', Ph.D. Centre for Development Studies, Thiruvananthapuram.

Rajasekharan, Tottam, (1991): *Udyogaparvam* (Service Memoir), Thiruvananthapuram.

Rao, Mohan (2004): *From Population Control to Reproductive Health: Malthusian Arithmetic*, Sage Publications, New Delhi.

Reidmann, Agnes. (1993): *Science that Colonizes: A Critique of Fertility Studies in Africa*, Temple University Press, Philadelphia.

Riley, Denise. (1995): *'Am I that Name?' Feminism and the Category of 'Women' in History*, University of Minnesota Press, Minnesota.

Row, T. Madava. (1889): *Hints on the Training of Native Children*, C. M.S. Press, Kottayam.

Sanoo, M.K. (1989): *Sahodaran K. Ayyappan* (biography), D.C Books, Kottayam.

——, (2002): *Yuktivaadi M.C. Joseph* (biography), Department of Cultural Publications, Government of Kerala, Thiruvananthapuram.

Saradamoni, K. (1999): *Matriliny Transformed: Family, Law and Ideology in Twentieth Century Travancore*, Sage Publications and Altamira Press, New Delhi.

Sastry, Velupillai.M.R. (1948): *Purogamanasahitya 'Kolahalam'* (The 'Furore' of Progressive Literature), Educational Supplies Depot, Thiruvananthapuram.

Schenk-Sandbergen, Loes. (1988): *Poverty and Survival: Kudumbi Female Domestic Servants and Their Households in Alleppey (Kerala)*, Manohar, New Delhi.

Singh, Jitendra. (1959): *Communist Rule in Kerala*, Diwan Chand India Information Centre, New Delhi.

Souvenir of the Kerala Catholic Regional Seminar, Aluva, December 1969.

Souvenir of the Fifteenth Haindava Mahasammelanam, Haindava Sevaka Sanghom, Thiruvananthapuram, 1952.

Sreekumar, Sharmila. (2001): 'Scripting Lives: Narratives by Dominant Women in a Southern State', PhD thesis submitted to Hyderabad Central University, Hyderabad.

State Planning Board (1969): *The Fourth Five-Year Plan 1969–1974: A Draft Outline*, Government of Kerala, Thiruvananthapuram.

Stein, D. (1995): *People Who Count: Population and Politics, Women and Children*, Earthscan, London.

Sukumaran, T.P. (1987): *Niroopakanaya Kesari*, D.C Books, Kottayam.

Symonds.R and M.Carder (1973): *The United Nations and the Population Question 1945–60*, Sussex University Press, London.

Teitelbaum, M.S, and J.M. Winter (1985): *The Fear of Population Decline*, Academic Press, Orlando, Florida.

Tharakan, Kocheapen P.K. (1993) [1922]: *Balikasadanam* (novel), Kerala Sahitya Akademi, Thrissur.

Tharakan, K.J.M. (1956): *Naveena Prasnangal* (Modern Problems), Kottayam.

Tharamangalam, Joseph, (1981): *Agrarian Class Conflict: The Political Mobilisation of Agricultural Labourers of Kuttanad, South India,* University of British Columbia Press, Vancouver.

Thomas, C.J. (1948): *Matavam Communisavum* (Religion and Communism), Kottayam.

van der Werff, Peter (1992): *Modern Poverty: The Culture of Distribution and Structural Unemployment in the Foothills of Kerala,* Manohar, New Delhi.

Varghese, K.E. (1981): *Slow Flows the Pampa: Socio-Economic Change in a Kuttanad Village in Kerala,* Concept Publishers, New Delhi.

——, (1986): *Socio-Economic Change in Kerala*, Ashish Publishing House, New Delhi.

Varma, P.K. Rajaraja (1969): *Kunjiyammayude Chintakal* (Kunjiyamma's Thoughts) (humorous essays), Rashmi Publications, Calcutta.

Vijayan, A., and J. Sandhya, (2004): *Gender and Decentralized Planning, Kerala, India*, SAKHI Women's Resource Centre, Thiruvananthapuram.

Weeks, Jeffrey (1981): *Sex, Politics, and Society: The Regulation of Sexuality since 1800*, Longman, London, New York.

Yesudas, R.N. (1975) *The People's Revolt in Travancore: A Backward Caste Movement for Social Freedom,* Kerala Historical Society, Thiruvananthapuram.

Zachariah, K.C, S. Irudaya Rajan, P.S. Sarma, K. Navaneetham, P.S. Gopinathan Nair, and U.S. Mishra (1994): *Demographic Transition in Kerala in the 1980s*, Centre for Development Studies, Thiruvananthapuram.

Zachariah, M. and R. Sooryamoorthy (1994): *Science for Social Revolution? Achievements and Dilemmas of a Development Movement: The Kerala Sastra Sahitya Parishad,* Zed Books, London.

Articles

Abraham, V.V., 'Adhyapakanmarum Manassastravum' (Teachers and Psychology), *MM Weekly,* 50, 11, 31 Oct. 1948, 14–16.

Accampo, Elinor A., 'The Gendered Nature of Contraception in France: Neo Malthusianism 1900–1920', *Journal of Interdisciplinary History,* 34,2, 2003, 35–62.

Ahluwalia, Sanjam, 'Demographic Rhetoric and Sexual Surveillance: Indian Middle Class Advocates of Birth Control, 1877–1947', paper presented at the Sixth Women in Asia Conference, Australian National University, Canberra, 2001.

Aiya, V. Nagam, Speech at Opening Ceremony of the Agricultural and Industrial Exhibition at Oachira, 14 June 1909, Thiruvananthapuram, Goverment Press.

Aiyar, K. Narayana, 'Balaramapuram Camp', *Kerala Kaumudi,* 15 May 1968, 3–4.

Alexander, V.K., 'Akarana Bhayam' (Unreasonable Fear), *Malayala Manorama Weekly,* 50 2, 29 Aug. 1948, 25–6.

Ali, Kamran, Asdar, 'Myths, Lies and Impotence: Structural Adjustment and Male Voice in Egypt', *Comparative Studies of South Asia, Africa and the Middle-East*, 23, 1, 2003, 321–34.

Ali, P.Muhammed, 'Muslim Leaginte Utkandha' (The Anxiety of the Muslim League), *Matrubhumi,* 13 Oct. 1967, 4.

Ambady, B.M., 'Santripta Kutumbam' (The Contented Family), *Kerala Kaumudi,* 12 July 1970, 5.

Amma, Kaveri, 'Nammude Pradhanappetta Chumatalakal' (Our Chief Responsibilities), *Malayala Manorama,* 10 Oct. 1925, 3.

Amma, Kochattil Kalyanikutty [Mrs C. Kuttan Nair], 'Swatantryavadikalaya Adhunika Matakkanmar' (Modern Mothers Who Are Votaries of Freedom), *Mahila,* 11, 2, 1931, 47–52.

Amma, C.K. Lakshmikutty, 'Janaperuppavum Vivahaprayavum' (Population Increase and the Age of Marriage), *Malayalarajyam,* 26 Aug. 1967, 3.

Amma, O.K. Madhavi, 'Kutumbasanvidhanam' (FP), *Matrubhumi,* 30 June 1971, 7.

Amma, E.N. Meenakshi, 'Vanitalokam' (Women's World), *M.N. Nair Masika,* 1,2, 1936, 122–6.

——, 'Vanitalokam' (Women's World), *M.N.Nair Masika,* vol. 3, 9/10, 1938, 464–5.

Amma, Saraswati, K., 'Jeevitarahasyangale Patti' (On the Secrets of Life), *Purushanmarillatta Lokam*, (Kottayam: Sahitya Pravartaka Sahakarana Sangham), 1958, 44–7.

Anandhi, S., 'Reproductive Bodies and Regulated Sexuality: Birth Control Debates in Early Twentieth Century Tamil Nadu,' *in* Mary E. John and Janaki Nair (eds.), *A Question of Silence? The Sexual Economies of Modern India*, (New Delhi: Kali for Women, 1988) 139–66.

Antarjanam, Lalitambika, N., 'Mulappalinte Manam' (The Scent of Breast-Milk) [1937], in *Agnipushpangal*, (Kottayam: Sahitya Pravartaka Sahakarana Sangham, 1973), 32–40.

Asad, Talal, 'Conscripts of Western Civilisation', *in* Christine Gailey (ed.), *Dialectical Anthropology: Essays in Honor of Stanley Diamond, vol. 1, Civilization in Crisis* (Gainseville: University of Florida, 1992), 332–40.

Awaya, Toshie, 'Women in the Nambutiri 'Caste' Movemen', *in* T. Mizushima and H. Yanagisawa (eds.), *History and Society in South India*, (Tokyo: Tokyo University of Foreign Studies, 1996), 47–57.

Ayappan, Parvati, 'Jeevitanilavaravum Swabhavaroopeekaranavum' (Standard of Life and the Formation of Character), *Kerala Kaumudi*, 22 July 1971, 5.

Babu, P.R.R., 'Pottitterikkunna Janasankhyayude Velluvili' (The Challenge of Exploding Population), *Malayala Manorama*, 30 April 1961, *I*.

Balakrishnan, Padmini, 'Kutumbajeevitam Enthinu? Engane?' (Family Life: For what? How?), *Matrubhumi Weekly* 41,16, 7July 1963, 29.

Basu, Alaka M., 'Birth Control by Assetless Workers in Kerala: The Possibility of a Poverty Induced Fertility Transition', *Development and Change* 17,2, 1986, 265–82.

Beasley, C, and C. Bacchi, 'Citizen Bodies: Embodying Citizen: A Feminist Analysis', *International Feminist Journal of Politics* 2, 3, 2000, 337–58.

Beevi, M. Nessimunnissa, 'An Evaluation of Family Welfare Programme *in* Kerala, India',in G.N. Rao (ed.), *Family*

Planning: The Afro-Asian Scenarios, Research Monograph Series vol. 5 Thiruvananthapuram, Centre for Development Studies, 1999, 231–42.

Beevi, Subaida, 'Udyogasthayaya Matavu Kutumbattinu Shapamo?' (The Officer- Mother: A Curse to the Family?), *Malayala Manorama* 23 Oct. 1969, 7.

Bhat, P.M, and S. Irudaya Rajan, 'Demographic Transition in Kerala Revisited', *Economic and Political Weekly,* xxv, 35–6, 1990, 1957–80.

Bledsoe, Caroline H., Allan H. Hill, Umberto D'Alessandro, Patricia Langerock, 'Constructing Natural Fertility: The Use of Western Contraceptive Technologies in Rural Gambia', *Population and Development Review,* 20,1, 1994, 81–113.

Buchanan, Francis, [1807] (1988), *A Journey from Madras Through Mysore, Canara and Malabar* vol. ii, New Delhi, Asia Educational Services.

Burchell, Graham, C. Gordon, P. Miller (eds.). *The Foucault Effect: Studies in Governmentality*, Chicago, Chicago University Press and Harvester Press, 1991.

Caldwell, J.C., 'Routes to Low Mortality in Poor Countries', *Population and Development Review,* 12, 2, 1986, 175–200.

Caldwell, J.C., Bruce Caldwell, and Pat Caldwell, 'Anthropology and Demography: The Mutual Reinforcement of Speculation and Research', *Current Anthropology,* xxviii, 1978, 25–34.

Carter, Anthony T., 'Does Culture Matter? The Case of the Demographic Transition', *Historical Methods,* xxi, 1988, 164–9.

Chacko, I.C., 'Krishivikasanam; Pambapaddhatikalum Mattu Paddhatikalum' (Agricultural Development: The Pampa and Other Projects), *Nazrani Deepika* 11 May 1949, 1.

Chacko, P.T., 'Kritrimasantananiyantranam'(Artificial Contraception), *Deepika Weekly* 5, 8, 1952, 3–10.

Chacko, P.T., 'Kutumba Samvidhanam: Kutumbathinte Adiverukal' (Family Planning—The Roots of the Family), *Nazrani Deepika,* 26 April 1959.

Chandy, Anna [1929], 'Streeswatantryathe Patti' (On Women's Independence), *in* J. Devika (ed. and trans.), *Her-Self: Early*

Writings on Gender by Malayali Women 1898–1938, Kolkata, Stree, 2005, 113–29.

——, 'Daurbalyabodham' (A Sense of Weakness), *Malayala Manorama* Annual Number, 1935, 14–15.

Chandrasekhar, S., 'A Note on Kerala's Population Problems', *Population Review* 10, 1, Jan. 1966, 68–71.

Chinnamma, K [1912] 2005, 'The Place of Women in Education', *in* J. Devika (ed.), *Her-Self: Early Writings on Gender by Malayali Women 1898–1938*, Kolkata, Stree, 29–36.

Cheriyan, Gracy, 'Akattum Purattum Modiyulla Veedu' (A House Splendid Inside and Outside), *Malayala Manorama* 27 Nov. 1970: 6.

Cook, Hera, 'The English Sexual Revolution: Technology and Social Change', *History Workshop Journal,* 59, 2005, 109–28.

Damodaran, N.K., 'Parishuddha Ezhavan, Chettatta Ezhavan', *Kerala Kaumudi* 4 Aug. 1968, 4.

Daniels, Cynthia R., and Janet Golden, 'Procreative Compounds: Popular Eugenics, Artificial Insemination and the Rise of the American Sperm Banking Industry', *Journal of Social History,* 38, 1, 2000, 5–27.

Das Gupta, Monica, "Libertié", "Egalité", Fraternité: Exploring the Role of Governance in Fertility Decline', *Journal of Development Studies,* 35, 5, 1999, 1–25.

Deshpande, Satish, 'Imagined Economies: Styles of Nation Building in Twentieth Century India', *Journal of Arts and Ideas,* nos. 25–6, 1993, 5–35.

Devadas, M.S., 'Premavum Purogamanasahityavum' (Romantic Love and Progressive Literature', in *Tiranhedutta Prabandhangal* (Selected Essays), Thrissur, Kerala Sahitya Akademi, 28–82.

Devi, V. Subhadra, 'Bharyayaya Udyogastaye Patti' (About the Employed Wife), *Kerala Kaumudi,* 10 March 1969, 6.

Devika, J., 'Possibilities in Ecofeminist Politics for Contemporary Kerala: A Note for Discussion', *Samyukta* 2, 2, 2002, 270–7.

——, 'Beyond *Kulina* and *Kulata*: The Critique of Gender Difference in the Writings of K. Saraswati Amma', *Indian Journal of Gender Studies,* 10, 2, 2003, 201–28.

——, 'The Idea of Being Malayali: The *Aikyakeralam* Movement of Mid-twentieth Century', paper presented at seminar on 'Recent Trends in South Indian Studies: Towards a Synthesis', MIDS, Chennai, 9–11, Dec. 2004.

——, 'The Aesthetic Woman: Re-forming Female Bodies and Minds in Early Twentieth Century Keralam', *Modern Asian Studies,* 39, 2, 2005, 461–88.

——, 'Negotiating Women's Space: Public Debates on Gender in Early Modern Kerala', India', *Inter-Asia Cultural Studies,* 7, 1, 2006, 43–61.

——, 'Housewife, Sex-Worker, and Re-former: Controversies over Women Writing Their Lives in Kerala', *Economic and Political Weekly*, xli, 17, 29 April 2006 (a).

Dowbiggin, Ian, 'A Rational Coalition: Euthanasia, Eugenics and Birth Control in Americal, 1940–1970', *Journal of Policy History,* 14, 3, 2002, 223–60.

Eapen, Mridul, 'Gender and Governance: Reviewing Kerala's Five-Year Plans', paper presented at the workshop on Gender and Governance, Bangalore, Aug. 2000.

Fischer, Dana, and Jessica F. Green, 'Understanding Disenfranchisement: Civil Society and Developing Countries' Influence and Participation in Global Governance for Sustainable Development', *Global Environmental Politics*, 43, 2004, 65–84.

Foucault, Michel, 'Politics and Reason', *Politics, Philosophy, Culture: Interviews and Other Writings 1977–1984*, London, Routledge, 1988, 57–85.

Folbre, N., 'Patriarchy and Fertility Decisions', *in* P. Demeny and G. Mc Nicoll (eds), *The Earthscan Reader on Population and Development*, Earthscan, London, 1998, 121–42.

Fraser, Arvonne S., 'Becoming Human: The Origin and Development of Women's Human Rights', *Human Rights Quarterly,* 21, 4, 1999, 853–906.

Gangadharan, M. 'Keraleeyata' [1974], in *Anveshanam, Asvadanam*, Kottayam, Sahitya Pravartaka Sahakarana Sangham, 1980, 32–44.

Goody, Jack, 'Globalisation, Population and Ecology', paper presented at the International Conference on Theoretical Topics in Ecological Economics, Trieste, Italy, 10–12, February, 2003.

Gopalan, A.K., 'Aikyakeralam' (United Kerala), in *Sardar K.M. Panikkar Shastipoorthy Smarakam*, Publications Committee, Kottayam, 1954, 236–38.

Greenhalgh, Susan, 'Towards a Political Economy of Fertility: Anthropological Contributions', *Population and Development Review,* 16,1, 1990, 85–101.

Greenhalgh, Susan, and Jiali Li, 'Engendering Reproductive Policy and Practice in Peasant China: For a Feminist Demography of Reproduction', *Signs: Journal of Women in Culture and Society,* 20, 3, 1995, 601–37.

Hammel E.A., 'A Theory of Culture for Demography', *Population and Development Review* 16, 3, 1990, 455–85.

Handelsman, David J., 'Bridging the Gender Gap in Contraception: Another Hurdle Cleared', *The Medical Journal of Australia* 154, 1991, 230–3.

Harcourt, Wendy, 'Revisiting the Population Question', *in* K. Saunders (ed.), *Feminist Post-Development Thought: Rethinking Modernity, Post-colonialism and Representation,* London and New York, Zed Press, New Delhi, Zubaan Books, 2004, 283–97.

Hauck, Christina, 'Abortion and the Individual Talent', *ELH,* 70, 1, 2003, 223–66.

Issac, T.M. Thomas, 'Class Struggle and Structural Change in the Coir Mat and Matting Industry in Kerala', Working Paper no. 142, Thiruvananthapuram, Centre for Development Studies, 1982.

Ittman, Karl, 'Demography as Policy Science in the British Empire, 1918–1969', *Journal of Policy History,* 15, 4, 2003, 417–48.

Jacob, Annamma, 'Udyogastayaya Kutumbini' (The Employed Housewife), *Malayala Manorama,* 22 Oct. 1971, 6.

Jacob, J.J., 'Santananiyantranamo' (Birth Control?), *Nazrani Deepika* 17 June 1936, 8.

Jeffrey, Patricia, and Roger Jeffrey, 'Silver Bullet or Passing Fancy? Girls' Schooling and Population Policy', *in* Cecile Jackson and Ruth Pearson (eds.), *Feminist Visions of Development: Gender Analysis and Policy,* London, New York, Routledge, 239–58.

Jeffrey, Roger, and Alaka M. Basu, 'Schooling as Contraception?'

in Roger Jeffrey and Alaka M.Basu (eds.), *Girls' Schooling, Women's Autonomy and Fertility Change in South Asia*, Sage Publications and The Book Review Trust, New Delhi, 1996, 15–47.

Job, T.J., 'Russiayum Sadacharavum' (Russia and Morality), *Deepika Weekly,* 5, 13, 1952, 23–25.

John, Mary, E., 'Globalisation, Sexuality and the Visual Field: Issues and Non-Issues for a Cultural Critique', *in* Mary E. John and Janaki Nair (eds), *A Question of Silence? The Sexual Economies of Modern India,* New Delhi, Kali for Women, 1998, 368–96.

Johnston, J. (1996). '"Flexing Femininity": Female Body-Builders Refiguring "The Body"' *Gender, Place and Culture,* 3, 3, 1996, 327–40.

Joseph, Annamma, 'Bharya Udyogastayayal' (When the Wife is Employed), *Malayala Manorama,* 6 July 1969, 4.

Joseph, M.O., 'Jananniyantranaprasthanam' (The Birth Control Movement), *Nazrani Deepika,* 22 Dec. 1933, 8.

Kabir, M., 'Beyond Philanthropy: The Rockfeller Foundation's Public Health Intervention in Thiruvitamkoor, 1929–1939', Working Paper no. 350, Centre for Development Studies, Thiruvananthapuram, 2003.

Kaler, Amy, '"Who Has Told You to Do This Thing?" Towards a Feminist Interpretation of Contraceptive Diffusion in Rhodesia, 1970–1980', *Signs: Journal of Women in Culture and Society,* 25, 3, 2000, 677–704.

Kalyanikutty, P., 'Santanangalkkidayilulla Prayavyatyasam' (Age-difference between Children), *Kerala Kaumudi* 13 Dec. 1969,5.

Karunakaran, C.O., 'Kutumbasootrananttinte Pracharanam' (Propagating Family Planning), *Matrubhumi,* 15 July 1965, 5.

——, 'Kutumbasootrana Paddhati' (The Family Planning Programme), *Kerala Kaumudi,* 11March 1967, 2.

——, 'Bahujanam Kanenda Oru Chitram!' (A Film That People Must See), *Kerala Kaumudi,* 1 Oct. 1967a, 6.

——, 'Janaperuppa Niyantranattinu Niyamanushasanam Anupekshaneeyam' (Legal Enactment Necessary for Population Control), *Kerala Kaumudi,* 24 Sept. 1967 b, 5.

——, 'Kutumbasamvidhanam Avidayum Ividayum' (Family Planning, There and Here), *Kerala Kaumudi,* 18 May 1968, 2.

——, 'Hridayasoonyaraya Bharttakkanmar: Sahatapikkate Enthu Cheyyum', (Heartless Husbands: What Else To Do but Sympathize), *Kerala Kaumudi,* 4 Jan. 1970, 4.

Kambissery Karunakaran, 'Communisavum Communalisavum' (Communism and Communalism), *Prabhatam,* 1, 8, Jan. 1945, 1,12.

Karippaayi, Sankaran, 'Premavum Laingikasaktiyum' (Love and Sexual Energy), *Yuvakeralam,* 1, 1, 1939, 22–3.

Kesavadev, P., 'Janananiyantranam: Atu Daridryattinu Pariharamakumo?' (Birth Control: A Solution to Poverty?), *Matrubhumi Weekly,* 10, 44, 23, Jan. 1933, 24.

Kittay, Eva Feder, 'A Feminist Public Ethic of Care Meets the New Communitarian Family Policy', *Ethics,* 111,3, 2006, 523–47.

Kodoth, Praveena, 'Courting Legitimacy or Delegitimising Custom? Sexuality, Sambandham and Marriage in Late 19th Century Malabar', *Modern Asian Studies,* 35, 3, 2001, 349–84.

—— and Mridul Eapen, 'Looking Beyond Gender Parities: Gender Inequities of Some Dimensions of Well-Being in Kerala', *Economic and Political Weekly*, 40, 30, 2005, 3278–86.

——, 'Varante 'Vila' Uyarunnu: Vivahaalochanayum Lingadhikaaravum Keralattil' (The 'Price' of the Bridegroom Increases: Marriage Negotiations and Gender Power in Kerala'), *in* J. Devika (ed.), *Aanarashunaattile Kaazhchbhakal: Kerala Streepakshagaveshanatthil,* Thiruvananthapuram, Women's Imprint, 2006, 83–118.

Krishnan, T.N., 'Demographic Transition in Kerala: Facts and Factors', *Economic and Political Weekly,* 11, 31–3, 1976, 1203–24.

Kunhuraman, C.V. 'Janaperuppam' (Increase in Population) [1938], *in* Putupally Raghavan (comp.), *C.V. Kunhuramante Tiranhedutta Kritikal* (Selected Writings of C.V. Kunhuraman), Thiruvananthapuram, Kaumudi Public Relations, 2004, 172–4.

Kurian, Annamma, 'Jananniyantranavum Kutumbinikalum'

(Birth Control and Housewives), *Malayala Manorama,* 28 Nov. 1969, 6.

Kurien, Grace, 'Ernakulatte Kutumbasootrana Camp Oru Mahatbhutam' (The Ernakulam Camps: A Great Miracle), *Matrubhumi,* 25 July 1971, 4.

Kurup, G. Sankara, 'Samyukta Keralam' (c. 1949), 'Keralasamsthanam', *in* G. Sankara Kurup, *Geeyude Gadyalekhanangal* (Prose Writings of G. Sankara Kurup), Kottayam, Sahitya Pravartaka Sahakarana Sangham, 1977, 350–1; 370–8.

Kurup, R.S, and T.K. Mathen, 'Sterilisation as a Method of Family Limitation in Kerala State', *Population Review,* 10, 2, 1966, 61–8.

Kurup, R.S, J.T. Chirayath, N.V. George, 'The After-effects of Sterilisation', in *Sterilisation: Demographic Particulars and After-effects*, Thiruvananthapuram, Bureau of Economics and Statistics, Demographic Research Centre, 1978, 13–35.

Kuttappan, K. 'Kuttikalude Anveshanabuddhi' (The Inquisitiveness of Children), *Malayalarajyam Weekly,* 12 Dec. 1965, 16–18.

Leiten, G.K., 'The Human Development Puzzle in Kerala', *Journal of Contemporary Asia,* 32, 1, 2002, 47–67.

Levin, Elise C., 'Women's Childbearing Decisions in Guinea: Life Course Perspectives and Historical Change', *Africa Today* 47,3/4, 2000, 63–81.

Lilly, C.K. 'Bharyayaya Udyogasta' (The Working Woman Who is Also a Wife), *Kerala Kaumudi,* 3 March 1968, 4.

Lingam, Lakshmi, 'Women, Population and the Development Question', *Economic and Political Weekly,* 15, Jan. 1994, 85.

'M', 'Ernakulatte Kootavasectomy' (Mass Sterilization at Ernakulam), *Matrubhumi,* 26 July 1971, 3.

'M', 'Kritrimasantananiyantranam Streetvathinu Orapamanam' (Artificial Contraception an Insult to Womanhood), *Nazrani Deepika,* 2 Oct. 1960, 5.

Main, Gloria L., 'Rocking the Cradle: Downsizing the New England Family', *Journal of Interdisciplinary History,* 37, 1, 2006, 35–58.

'Malayalikal Marunnattil' (Malayalis Abroad) [author not

mentioned], *Kerala Kaumudi,* 26 Sept. 1968, 2.

Maliakkal, Joseph, 'Catholica Conference: Oru Tiruttal' (Catholic Conference: A Clarification), *Nazrani Deepika,* 15 June 1949, 3.

Mamdani, Mahmood, 'The Ideology of Population Control', *Economic and Political Weekly,* Annual no. Aug. 1976, 1141–8.

Mathen, George [1865], 'Marumakkathayattalulla Doshangal' (The Evils of Matriliny), *Vidyasangraham: The Cottayam College Quarterly Magazine* 1 (5) 1865: rpt. Benjamin Bailey Research Centre, *Vidyasangraham July 1864–April 1866*; Reprinted, Kottayam, CMS College, 1993, 347–8.

Mathias, Louis, 'Santananiyantranam', *Deepika Weekly,* 4, 1, 1951, 16–20.

McDaniels, Susan, 'Towards a Synthesis of Feminist and Demographic Perspectives on Fertility', *Sociological Quarterly,* 37, 1, 1996, 83–104.

Meldrum, Marcia L., '"Simple Methods" and "Determined Contraceptors": The Statistical Evaluation of Fertility Control 1957–1968', *Bulletin of the History of Medicine,* 70, 2, 1996, 266–95.

Menon, C, Achyuta, 'Soviet Naadu: Oru Putiya Lokam' (The Land of the Soviets) [1942], in *C. Achyuta Menonte Sampoorna Kritikal,* vol. iv (The Collected Works of C. Achyuta Menon), Thiruvananthapuram, Prabhat Publishers, 2003, 23–253.

Menon, Bindu M., 'Shadow Lines: Cinema and Social Space in Early 20th Century Thiruvithamkoor', paper Presented at the SARAI Student Fellowship workshop, CSDS, New Delhi, 26 Aug. 2005.

Menon, Janardana, Kunnathu, [1934], 'Abhinavachaturvarnyam' (Modern Caste-Order) *Lekhavati,* Kozhikode, Prakashakaumudi Printing, 1955, 105–15.

Menon, G. Raman, 'Tiruvitamkoorile Uppum Chorum' (The Salt and Rice in Travancore), *Nazrani Deepika,* 14 Aug. 1929,1.

Menon, Puttezhattu Raman, [1955], 'Laingika Pathanam'(Sex-Education), in *Arivulla Ajnanikal,* Kottayam, Sahitya Pravartaka Sahakarana Sangham, 1970, 11–17.

——, [1955], 'Janapperuppavum Bhakshanakshamavum' (Population Increase and Food Shortage), in *Arivulla Ajnanikal,*

Kottayam, Sahitya Pravartaka Sahakarana Sangham, 1970, 72–92.

——, 'Onam!!' in *Parihasattiloote*, Kottayam, Sahitya Pravartaka Sahakarana Sangham, 1969, 1–29.

——, 'Kritrima Ari' (Artificial Rice) in *Parihasattiloote*, Kottayam, Sahitya Pravartaka Sahakarana Sangham, 1969, 228–38.

——, 'Samyamanavum Samskaravum'(Self-Control and Culture), in P.K. Narayana Pillai (ed.), *Gadyakairali,* part iv, Thiruvananthapuram, University of Kerala, 1969, 45–54.

Mishra, Udaya S., 'Women's Health in Kerala: Illusions and Realities', paper presented at the workshop 'Women's Health in Kerala: Issues and Challenges', SAKHI, Thiruvananthapuram, 5–6 May 2006.

Morrison, Barrie M., 'The Embourgeoisment of the Kerala Farmer', *Modern Asian Studies,* 31,1, 61–87, 1997.

Moonjoli, Thomas, 'Jananiyantrana Bhramam' (The Folly of Birth Control), *Nazrani Deepika,* 4 June 1929, 5.

Mrinalini, 'Kalyanam Kaliyalla' (Marriage is no Play), *Matrubhumi Weekly,* 41, 10, 26, May 1963, 28.

'M.S.' (pseudonym), 'Kutumbajeevitam', *Malayala Manorama Weekly,* 50,120, Nov. 1948, 19–22.

Nadkarni, M.V., 'Overpopulation and the Rural Poor', *Economic and Political Weekly,* Annual Number, 1976, 1163–73.

Nair, A.P.G., 'Takarunna Keralam' (Disintegrating Keralam), *Jayakeralam,* November 1958, 9.

Nair, M.S. Bhaskaran, 'Kutumbasootranam Vandhyamkaranam Matram Avarutu'(FP Must Not Be Sterilization Alone), *Matrubhoomi,* 8 June 1971,4.

Nair, M.N.Govindan, see 'Sadhukkal Bharttakkanmar' (Poor Husbands) [1936], *in* M.N. Govindan Nair, *Gopivilasam,* Kottayam, 1950, 50–6.

Nair, P.M., 'Santananiyantranam' (Contraception), *Arogyam,* Special Issue 1932, 76–89.

Nair, P. R.G., 'Decline in Birth Rate in Kerala: A Hypothesis About the Interrelationship Between Demographic Variables, Health Services and Education', *Economic and Political Weekly,* Annual Number, 1974, 323–36.

Nair, M. Gopalakrishnan, (Comp.), *Sahityapanchananante Kritikal,* vol. iii: *Smaranayum Samskaravum* (Collected Works of 'Sahityapanchananan' P.K. Narayana Pillai), Thiruvananthapuram, State Institute of Languages, 1995, 178–80.

Nair, Govindankutty, Ullattil, 'Manushyavargathinte Bhavi' (The Future of Humanity) in *Vicharadhara*, Kozhikode, P.K. Brothers, 1962, 16–21.

Nair, E. A. Karunakaran, 'Bhroonahatya Papamo?'(Is Abortion a Sin?) in *Buddhimanaya Putran Janikkan*, Kottayam, Sahitya Pravartaka Sahakarana Sangham, 1984, 5–9.

Nair, K.G. Kesavan, 'Manasinte Atbudhasaktikal' (The Wondrous Powers of the Mind), serialized in *Malayalarajyam Weekly*, Oct.–Nov. 1956.

Nambiar, P.Sankaran, Keralabhyudayam', *Sahityanishkudam* [essays], Kozhikode, Deccan Publishing House, 1943, 158–65.

Nambutiripad, Kanippayyur Sankaran, 'Dambathyabandham' (Conjugal Relations), *Unny Nambutiri,* 7,7, 1925, 423–32.

Nambutiripad, E.M.S., 'Keralattile Samudayasanghatanakal: Avayodu Perumarendatengane?' [1936](Community Movements in Keralam: How to Approach Them?), rpt *in* P. Govinda Pillai (ed.) *EMS Sampoorna Kritikal* vol. ii 1946–7 [Collected Works], Thiruvananthapuram, Chinta Publications, 1999, 86–94.

——, 'Kazhinja 30 Varsham Chatuppu: Innu Punchiri Tookum Pachappadam' [1944] (Swamp for the Past 30 Years: Today a Green Field Beaming Bright) in P. Govinda Pillai (ed.), *E.M.S. Sampoorna Kritikal* 1952–3, Thiruvananthapuram, Chinta Publication, 2000, 84–6.

——, *Nambutiriye Manushyanakkan* (To Make Man out of the Nambutiri), Desabhimani, 1945.

——, 'Ongallur Prasangattinu Shesham' (1946) (After the Speech at Ongallur), rept *in* P. Govinda Pillai (ed.), *EMS Sampoorna Kritikal,* vol. vii [Collected Works] 1946–7, Thiruvananthapuram, Chinta Publications, 1999, 228–34.

——, 'Onnekalkoti Malayalikal' (1946b) (A Crore and a Quarter Malayalis), rptd *in* P. Govinda Pillai (ed.), *EMS Sampoorna Kritikal,* vol. vi, 1946–7, Thiruvananthapuram, Chinta Publications, 1999, 288–347.

——, 'Marxisavum Sanmargabodhavum' [1949] (Marxism and Morality), *in* P. Govinda Pillai (ed.), *EMS: Sampoorna Kritikal* vol. viii, 1947–9, Thiruvananthapuram, Chinta Publications, 1999, 282–96.

——, 'A. Balakrishna Pillai: Bourgeois Panditamoodhanmarute Uttamamatrka' [1949] (A. Balakrishna Pillai: An Ideal Model for Senseless Bourgeois Scholars), in P. Govinda Pillai (ed.), *EMS: Sampoorna Kritikal,* vol. viii, 1947–9, Thiruvananthapuram, Chinta Publications, 1999, 336–45.

——, 'Aikyakeralasatrukkalute Turuppucheetu: Bhakhyakkammi' [1953] (The Ace held by Enemies of United Keralam: Food Deficit) from P. Govinda Pillai (ed.), *E.M.S. Sampoorna Kritikal,* vol. xiv, March 1953–Feb. 1954, Thiruvananthapuram, Chinta Publications, 2000, 314–18.

——, *Keralathile Sambattika Prasnangal* (Economic Problems of Keralam), Thiruvananthapuram, Prabhatam Publications, 1956.

——, 'Planningum Vyavasayavatkaranavum' (Planning and Industrialization), *Janayugam Weekly,* Annual Number, 1963, 16–28.

Namboodiri, D.D. (1999),' Caste and Social Change in Colonial Kerala', *in* P.J. Cheriyan (ed.), *Perspectives on Kerala History*, Kerala State Gazetteers vol. ii, Thiruvananthapuram, Government of Kerala, 426–55.

Narayanan, Dhanya, 'Kutumbam Innale, Innu, Nale' (The Family: Yesterday, Today, Tomorrow), *Malayala Manorama,* 19 Sept. 1969, 6.

Narayanan, K.R., 'Janasankhya Ingane Perukiyal!' (If Population Grows Like This!), *Malayala Manorama,* Sunday Supplement, 14 Aug. 1966, I.

Noujain, Elie Georges, 'History as Geneology: An Exploration of Foucault's Approach to History', *Philosophy* (Suppl.), 21, 1986–7, 157–74.

Nelson, Jennifer A., 'Abortions under Community Control: Feminism, Nationalism and the Politics of Reproduction among New York City's Young Lords', *Journal of Women's History,* 13, 1, 2001, 157–80.

Nellayi, George, 'Communist Vyavastayil Kutumbe

Bhadrataikkulla Sthanam' (The Place of Family Stability Within the Communist System), *Nazrani Deepika Weekly*, 5, 27, 1952, 16–17.

Nenminimangalam, Parvati, 'Streetvam' (Womanliness), *Stree*, 1, 1, 1933, 15–16.

Newland, Lynda, 'The Deployment of the Prosperous Family: Family Planning in West Java', *National Women's Studies Association Journal*, 13, 3, 2001, 22–48.

Nieuwenhuys, Olga, 'Emancipation for Survival: Access to Land and Labour of Thandans in Kerala', *Modern Asian Studies*, 25, 3, 1991, 599–619.

'Nireekshakan' (pseudonym), 'Santananiyantranam: Atu Sweekaryamano?' (Birth control: Is It Acceptable?), *Nazrani Deepika*, 7 Jan. 1936, 2.

Obermeyer, C.M., 'Reproductive Choices in Islam: Gender and State in Iran and Tunisia', *Studies in Family Planning*, 25, 1, 1994, 41–51.

Oudshoorn, Nelly, 'Astronauts in the Sperm World', *Men and Masculinities*, 6, 4, 2004, 349–67.

Oommen, M.A., 'Dhanakaryacommissionum Keralavum' (The Finance Commission and Kerala), *Malayala Manorama*, Sunday Supplement, 8 Oct. 1961, i.

——, [1963] 'Agriculture in the Third Five Year-Plan: Some Sidelights from Kerala,' in *Essays on Kerala Economy*, New Delhi, Oxford University Press and India Book House, 1993, 34–44.

Oommen, M.I., 'Entu Vilayum Koduttu Janasankhya Niyantriche Teeru' (Population Should be Controlled at All Costs), *Malayala Manorama*, Sunday Supplement, 20 Feb. 1966, iii.

Ortiz-Ortega, Adriana, and Judith F. Helzner, 'Opening Windows to Gender: A Case Study in a Major International Population Agency, *Social Politics: A Journal of Gender, State and Society*, 10, 1, 2003, 129–52.

Panikar, K.K., 'Sanghatana Venamo?' (Do We Need Organization?), *Vivekodayam*, 20, 5, 1930, 177–79.

Panikker, Lalita Mohana, 'Streekalkku Oru Putiya Veekshanam Avashyam' (Women Need a New Vision), *Kerala Kaumudi*, 16 March 1969, 4.

Parambil, Jose Vakayil, 'Janananiyantranam' (Birth Control), *Nazrani Deepika Weekly,* 5, 46, 1952, 17–19.

Pennammabhayi, 'Our Economic Position and Women', *in* J. Devika (ed.), *Her-Self: Early Writings on Gender by Malayalee Women,* Kolkata, Stree, 2005, 154–57.

Petersen, W., 'Urban Policies in Africa and Asia', *Population Review,* 10, 1, 1966, 24–35.

Pillai, Kesari A. Balakrishna, 'Malayaliyude Bhavi', P. Krishnan Nair (Comp.), *Gadyakusumavali,* Part II, Thiruvananthapuram, 1934, 23–9.

Pillai, Changampuzha Krishna, 'Sahitya Chintakal' in *Purogamana Sahityam Enthinu*? Kottayam, Sahitya Pravartaka Sahakarana Sangham, 1953, 71–2.

Pillai, R. Easwara, 'Chila Samudaya Chintakal—Nammude Samudayashakti' (Some Thoughts on Community: The Strength of Our Community), *Service* 5,1, 1926, 9–13.

——, 'Uttaravaditvattinte Kaimattam' (Transfer of Responsibility), *Mahila,* 16, 1, 1936, 200–5.

Pillai, Paravur K. Gopala, 'Chila Dambatyasastra Rahasyangal' (Some Secrets of Conjugal Science), *Kutumbapatrika,* 2, 2, 1934, 10–12.

Pillai, Malloor Govinda, 'Aikyakeralavum Keralasarvakalashalayum,' *in* K.Sivarama Panikkar, *Malloor: Oru Matruka Jeevitam* [biography], Thiruvananthapuram, 1954, 99–106.

Pillai, Kuttippuzha Krishna, 'Streekalude Paratantryam' [1941] (The Unfreedom of Women), in *Kuttippuzhayute Prabandhangal* vol. iii (Essays of Kuttippuzha), Thrissur, Kerala Sahitya Akademi, 1990, 13–14.

——, 'Russiayile Streekal' [1944] (Women of Russia), in *Kuttippuzhayute Prabandhangal,* vol. iii (Essays of Kuttippuzha), Thrissur, Kerala Sahitya Akademi, 1990, 54–6.

——, 'Janananiyantranam' (1962), in *Kuttippuzhayute Prabandhangal,* vol iii (Essays of Kuttippuzha), Thrissur, Kerala Sahitya Akademi, 1990, 121–5.

——, 'Dambatya Jeevitattile Sambattika Khatakam' (The Financial Factor in Married Life) [1965], *Kuttippuzhayute Prabandhangal* vol. iii (Essays of Kuttippuzha), Thrissur, Kerala Sahitya Akademi, 1990, 152–5.

Pillai, K.S., 'Nammude Janasankyayum Bhakshyaprasnavum'(Our Population and the Food Crisis), *Malayalarajyam,* 8 Jan. 1967, 4.

Pillai, Changanashery Parameshwaran 'Janavardhana' (Increase in Population), *Kutumbapatrika,* 2, 7, 1934, 8.

Pillai, Soma Krishna, 'Veetammamar Vazhittiruvil' (Housewives at Crossroads), *Malayala Manorama,* 10 Oct. 1969, 6.

Posner, Richard A., 'Orwell Versus Huxley: Economics, Technology, Privacy, and Satire', *Philosophy and Literature,* 24 (1), 2000, 1–33.

Pothuvalsyar, Ambady Narayani, 'Ambalavasi Samudayam' (The Ambalavasi Community), *Yuvachaitanyam* 1, 1 Oct.–Nov. 1933, 46–7.

Poovey, M., 'The Abortion Question and the Death of Man,' *in* J. Butler and J. Scott (eds.), *Feminists Theorise the Political,* London, Routledge, 1992, 239–56.

Qadeer, I., 'Our Historical Legacy in Maternal and Child Health Programmes', *in* M. Krishna Raj, R. M. Sudarshan, Abusaleh Shariff (eds.), *Gender, Population and Development,* New Delhi, Oxford University Press, 1998, 267–90.

Raja, C. Unny, 'Kerala Samsthanappiraviyute Prasnangal', *Janayugam,* Onam Special Number, 1956.

Rajan S. Irudaya, Mala Ramanathan, U.S. Mishra, 'Female Autonomy and Reproductive Behaviour *in* Kerala', in Roger Jeffreys and Alaka M. Basu (eds.), *Girls' Schooling, Women's Autonomy and Fertility Change in South Asia,* New Delhi, Sage Publications, 1996, 268–87.

Rajan, S. Irudaya, U.S. Mishra, and T.K. Vimala, 'Role of Abortion in the Fertility Transition in Kerala', *Demography India,* 29, 1, 2000, 75–84.

Ramaiyer, Kamala, 'Kutumbashreyassum Kutumbasootranavum' (Family Well Being and FP), *Malayala Manorama,* 18 Dec. 1959, 2.

Ramachandran, Sati, 'Udyogastakalaya Matakkalum

Kunhungalum'(Working Mothers and Children), *Kerala Kaumudi* 4 May 1970, 5.

Ramachandran, V.K. 'On Kerala's Development Achievements,' *in* J. Dreze and A. Sen (eds.), *Indian Development: Selected Regional Perspectives*, UN / WIDER, New Delhi, Oxford University Press, 1997, 205–35.

——, 'Kerala's Development Achievements and their Replicability,' *in* G. Parayil (ed.), *Kerala: The Development Experience*, London and New York, Zed Press, 2000, 88–115.

Ramanathan, Mala, T.R. Dilip and S. S. Padmadas, 'Quality of Care in Laparoscopic Sterilisation Camps: Observations from Kerala, India', *Reproductive Health Matters,* 3, 6, 1995, 84–93.

Ramakrishnan, E.V., 'Pattalakathakalile Rashtrasankalpam' (The Concept of the Nation in Army Stories), in *Vakkile Samooham*, Kottayam, D.C Books, 1997, 41–9.

Ramusack, Barbara. N. (1989), 'Embattled Advocates: The Debate over Birth Control in India, 1920–1940', *Journal of Women's History,* 1, 2, 1989, 34–64.

Rao, M.S.A. (1957), *Social Change in Malabar*, Bombay, Popular Prakashan.

Rao, N.B., and K.N.M. Raju. 'Population, Health and Family Planning,' *in* P.V. Shenoi (ed), *Contours of Social and Economic Development: Policy Issues,* New Delhi, Concept Publishers, 1997, 222–41.

Ratcliffe, J., 'Social Justice and Demographic Transition: Lessons from India's Kerala State', *International Journal of Health Services,* 8,1, 1978, 123–44.

Raveendran, N.K., 'Keralattile Streevimochanarashtreeyam: Charitraparamaya Oranveshanam' (Feminist Politics in Kerala: A Historical Enquiry), in K. Satchidanandan (ed.), *Streepadhanangal*, Bodhi Books, Kozhikode, n.d., 43–91.

Ravikumar, K.S. 'Introduction', *in* K.S. Ravikumar (ed.), *K. Saraswati Ammayude Sampoorna Kritikal* (The Complete Works of K. Saraswati Amma), Kottayam, D.C Books, i-ii.

Ravindran, Sundari T.K., 'Women and the Politics of Population and Development in India', *Reproductive Health Matters,* 1, 1993, 26–38.

Ruhl, L., 'Dilemmas of the Will: Uncertainty, Reproduction, and the Rhetoric of Control', *Signs,* 27, 3, 2002, 641–63.

Roach, Catherine, 'Loving Your Mother: On the Woman–Nature Relation', *Hypatia,* 6, 1, 1991, 56–60.

Robeyns, Ingrid, 'Sen's Capability Approach and Feminist Concerns', paper presented at the conference on Amartya Sen's Capabilities Approach, St Edmund's College, Cambridge, 5–7, June 2001.

Rose, Nikolas, 'Governing "Advanced" Liberal Democracies', *in* Andrew Barry, Thomas Osborne, Nikolas Rose (eds.), *Foucault and Political Reason: Liberalism, Neo-liberalism and Rationalities of Government,* London, UCL Press, 1996, 32–83.

Rose, Susan, 'Going too Far? Sex, Sin and Social Policy', *Social Forces,* 84, 2, 2005, 1207–32.

Sadasivan, M.P., 'Kutumbakshema Pakshacharanam' (Celebrating Family Planning Week), *Malayala Manorama,* 5 July 1970, iv.

Sahib, Seeti. [1958], 'Vargeeyatayum Desheeyatvavum' (Communalism and Nationalism), *in* Abu Siddique, *Seethi Sahib: Jeevacharitram,* Kozhikode, 1966, 208–15.

Sakamoto, Hiroko, 'The Cult of "Love and Eugenics" in May Fourth Movement Discourse', *Positions: East Asia Cultures Critique,* 12, 2, 2004, 329–76.

Sankaran, Tayattu, 'Bharateeyata', in *Balamani Amma Sashtipoorthy Smaranika,* Kozhikode, Publication Committee, 1969, 65–6.

[Author not mentioned], Santananiyantranam' (Birth Control), *Mahila,* vol. 12, 11–12, 1932, 373.

Saradamoni, K., 'Women, Reproduction and Work', *in* K. Saradamoni (ed.), *Finding the Household: Conceptual and Methodological Issues,* Women in the Household in Asia, 5, New Delhi, Sage Publications, 1992, 163–80.

Schneider, Peter, and Jane Schneider (1995), 'Coitus Interruptus and Family Respectability in Catholic Europe: A Sicilian Case Study', *in* Faye D. Ginsberg and Rayna Rapp (eds), *Conceiving the New World Order: The Global Politics of Reproduction,* Berkeley, University of California Press, 177–94.

Schoen, Johanna, 'Between Choice and Coercion: Women and the Politics of Sterilization in North Carolina, 1929–1975,

Journal of Women's History, 13, 1, 2001, 132–56.

Shapiro, Michael, J., 'Literary Production as a Politicising Practice', *Political Theory*, 12, 1984, 389–98.

Smith, Andrea, 'Beyond Pro-Choice Versus Pro-Life: Women of Color and Reproductive Justice', *National Women's Studies Association Journal,* 17, 1, 2005, 119–140.

Smith, Daniel Jordan. 'These Girls Today *Na War-O*: Premarital Sexuality and Modern Identity in Southeastern Nigeria', *Africa Today* 47, 3/4, 2000, 99–120.

Smith, James M., 'The Politics of Sexual Knowledge: The Origins of Ireland's Containment Culture and the Carrigan Report (1931)', *Journal of the History of Sexuality* 13, 2, 2004, 208–33.

Smyth, Ines., 'Gender Analysis of Family Planning: Beyond the 'feminist vs. Population Control Debate', *in* Cecile Jackson and Ruth Pearson (eds.), *Feminist Visions of Development: Gender Analysis and Policy,* London, Routledge, 1998, 217–38.

Sowmini, C.V. and P. Sankara Sarma, 'Reproductive Morbidity among Contraceptive Users: Need for Quality Services', *Journal of Family Welfare,* 50, 1, 2004, 31–7.

Sukumaran, P.K., 'Santananiyantranamo Sambattikasootranamo' (Birth Control or Economic Planning), *Janayugam Weekly,* Onam Special Issue, 1963, 14–23.

Sukumaran, Usha, 'Udyogastayaya Bharya: Oru Vishadeekaranam' (The Employed Wife: An Explanation), *Malayala Manorama,* 19 Nov. 1971, 3.

Szreter, C.S., 'The Idea of Demographic Transition and the Study of Fertility Change: A Critical Intellectual History', *Population and Development Review,* 19, 4, 1993, 659–702.

Szreter, C.S., R.A. Nye, and F. van Poppel, 'Fertility and Contraception during the Demographic Transition: Quantitative and Qualitative Approaches', *Journal of Interdisciplinary History,* 34, 2, 2003, 141–54.

Tampuran, L.A. Ravi Varma, 'Lokopakaramaya Oru Vidyabhyasakramam' (A System of Education Useful to Society), *Swadeshabhimani,* 3, 5–6, 1924–5, 217–22.

Tharakan, Michael P.K., 'Socio–Religious Reform Movements and Demand for Indications of Development: Thiruvitamkoor

1860–1930', *in* Alok Bhalla and Peter Burke (eds.), *Images of Rural India in the Twentieth Century*, New Delhi, Sterling Publishers, 1992, 134–52.

——, 'Land relations in Contemporary Keralam: A Survey' in V.K. Ramachandran, Madhura Swaminathan (eds.) *Agrarian Studies: Essays on Agrarian Relations in Less Developed Countries*, New Delhi, Tulika, 2000, 355–61.

Thomas, C.J., 'Veshavum Sadacharavum', in *Ivan Ente Priya Putran*, Kottayam, Sahitya Pravartaka Sahakarana Sangham, 1953, 19–25.

Thomas, P.J., 'Keralasamsthanam Enthinu?' (Why the State of Kerala?), in *Sardar K.M. Panikkar Shastipoorthy Smarakam*, Kozhikode, Publication Committee, 1954, 240–44.

——, 'Dandakaranya Paddhatiyum Keralavum' (Kerala and the Dandakaranya Project), *Malayala Manorama,* 17 Nov. 1960.

Thornton, Arland, 'The Developmental Paradigm, Reading History Sideways, and Family Change', *Demography,* 38, 4, 2001, 449–65.

Twine, Richard. T., 'Ma(r)king Essence: Ecofeminism and Embodiment', *Ethics and Environment,* 6, 2, 2001, 31–58.

Udayabhanu, A.P., 'Kutumbasootranam Oru Dharmam' (Family Planning: A Duty), *Malayala Manorama,* 15 July 1965,4.

——, 'Entoru Jeevitamanu Ningal Enikku Tannatu' (What a Life have You Given Me), *Matrubhumi* 19 Sept. 1967, 4.

——, 'Vasectomyum Jnanum' (Vasectomy and Me), *Matrubhumi,* 26 March 1970, 5.

University of Kerala, *Family Growth: Desires, Ideals and Achievement,* Department of Statistics, Thiruvananthapuram, 1965.

Vadakkan, Brother, 'Sa. Damodaran Sannadhanano?' (Is Comrade Damodaran Ready?), *Tozhilali,* 26 July 1953.

Varghese, Mathew, M., 'Population Growth and Economic Development in Kerala' in *Selected Studies in Population and Family Welfare Programme,* vol. iii, Thiruvananthapuram, Bureau of Economics and Statistics, 1983, 155–73.

Varma, Rama, 'Our Industrial Status', lecture delivered to the Trevandrum Debating Society, 26 Sept. 1864, C.M.S Press, Kottayam, 1874.

Varma, Rajaraja P.K., 'Vitamin E', in *President Kunji*, Kottayam, 1948.

Vasantan, S.K., 'Devinte Novel Shilpam,' *in* K.M. Tarakan (ed.), *Tulika Padavalakkiya Kesava Dev*, D.C Books, Kottayam, 1986, 11–16.

Velappan, Viji, 'Santushta Kutumbam: Adyam Tanne Adittara Paniyuka (The Happy Family: Build the Foundation First), *Malayala Manorama,* 12 June 1970, 6.

Velayudhan, Dr G. 'Enthanee Kutumbasamvidhanam?'(What is this Family Planning?), *Kerala Kaumudi,* 24 Sept. 1967, 5.

Velayudhan, Meera, 'Reform, Law and Gendered Identity', *in* M.A. Oommen (ed.), *Rethinking Development: Kerala's Development Experience* vol. i, Institute of Social Research and Concept Publishers, New Delhi, 1999, 60–72.

Warrier, M.R. Madhava, address to the Annual Conference of the *Prakriti Vaidya Samajam* (Association of Natural Healers), *Arogyam,* 2, 8/9,1925–6, 41–56.

Warrier, K.V. Sankara. 'Samudaya Parishkaranam: Ekeekaranam', *Swajanaranjini,* 1, 4, 1934, 132–6.

Wilson, Amrit, 'New World Order and the West's War on Population', *Economic and Political Weekly*, 20, Aug. 1994, 2202.

Wheeler, Leigh Ann, 'Rescuing Sex from Prudery and Prurience: American Women's Use of Sex Education as an Antidote to Obscenity, 1925–1932', *Journal of Women's History,* 12, 3, 2000, 173–95.

Zachariah, K.C., 'The Anomaly of the Fertility Decline in Kerala: A Field Investigation', Staff Working Paper no. 700, Washington D.C, World Bank, 1984.

——, 'The Syrian Christians of Kerala: Demographic and Socioeconomic Transition in the Twentieth Century', Working Paper no. 322, Thiruvananthapuram, Centre for Development Studies, 2001.